Healing Beyond Pills

Healing Beyond Pills

Exploring Holistic Therapies for Chronic Stress

Vivienne Mallory

Mindful Pages

Published in 2025

ISBN: 9789371774383 (PB)
ISBN: 9789371779098 (eBook)

Published by

Mindful Pages
Imprint of Alpha Editions LLC
312 W. 2nd St #1834
Casper, WY 82601, USA

Content

Introduction
The Unspoken Language of Stress: Rethinking the Root

Stress has slipped into our vocabulary with an unsettling ease—invoked as complaint, boast, or even proof of our engagement with modern life. We carry it like an invisible burden, sometimes flaunt it as a kind of grim credential. Yet what if the story we've been told about stress is incomplete? Suppose chronic stress is less a malfunction and more a message—a complex form of communication between body, mind, and spirit. This book begins with a quiet but radical proposal: chronic stress is not simply a disorder to be contained; it is a messenger, speaking in the dialect of tension, fatigue, disconnection, and dis-ease. It speaks for reasons that deserve our attention.

Behind the sleepless nights and inflamed joints, beyond the diagnoses and clinical language, there is something older than pathology. A call. A signal as ancient as human memory, drowned out by the hum of technology and the churn of productivity. Contrary to the popular framing, we are not merely passive recipients of life's pressures. We are creatures of rhythm, pattern, and deep memory. And when those inner patterns are broken—by speed, fragmentation, and the erosion of rest—the body does not simply absorb the blow. It remembers. It protests. It adapts, but at a cost.

The promise of *Healing Beyond Pills* is not that it will soothe you in the conventional way. This is not a book of quick fixes. You will not find lists for reorganising your schedule or neat strategies to trick the brain into docility. Instead, it offers something far rarer: a change of orientation. A turning towards the source rather than away from the symptoms. A fresh understanding of what stress is and what it means, met not with dread but with curiosity, respect, and care that is felt in the bones.

This epidemic of chronic stress is not only biological—it is cultural, ecological, existential. We are made to keep pace with systems that commodify health and monetise strain, then told our struggle is a personal failing. This is a narrow—and impoverished—view. Older medical traditions knew better. Long before modern biomedicine declared itself the authority, systems like Ayurveda, Traditional Chinese Medicine, Taoist practice, and naturopathy recognised that symptoms are not faults in the machinery, but signposts. A liver out of balance, a restless mind, a shallow breath—these were seen as meaningful, threads in a larger conversation.

Such traditions, grounded in observation and reverence, did not declare stress an adversary to be annihilated. They saw it as imbalance—an invitation home. This book draws from those lineages not to romanticise, but to reclaim what our transactional wellness culture has lost: context, connection, coherence.

Our journey here begins with listening—to the breath, to the body, to the unspoken stories lodged in both. Each chapter becomes a conversation with a different aspect of the stress experience. We'll explore how relentless speed erodes memory, how the nervous system is as much shaped by narrative as by stimulus, and how the body holds a quiet, often ignored wisdom. We will look again at what it means to rest, to nourish, to belong.

This is not a tidy manual. Think of it as a living map—part science, part philosophy, part excavation of what is most human. You will walk it rather than simply read it. The practices within are not instructions so much as invitations: to slow down, to remember what was once instinctive, to trust that healing comes from within when conditions are right.

The prevailing model of stress fails not for lack of tools but for lack of depth. It treats stress as a glitch in the system, isolated from meaning. It seeks to silence symptoms rather than understand them. Yet chronic stress has patterns; it often begins where we have drifted from ourselves—when our speed outruns our sense of purpose, when our duties consume our identity. These fractures cannot be medicated into oblivion forever. They need to be witnessed. They need realignment. They need the space to breathe.

This book is such a space.

It is a slow return to the self—not the self of slogans and self-improvement plans, but the ecological self, the storied self, the embodied self. It offers a critique—sometimes a sharp one—of the forces that profit from our alienation: the cult of productivity, the machinery of medical commerce, the hollow myth of radical independence. Healing here is not solitary. It is relational. Political. Ancestral. And it is unhurried.

You will meet in these pages healers who work through touch and rhythm, scientists who honour the sacred, patients who became their own medicine. You'll learn not only the mechanics of breath but the language it speaks. Not just how to support your digestion, but how to listen for the emotional currents that shape it. Not only how to rest, but how to reclaim rest as an act of quiet defiance.

The chapters are crafted to move from seeing stress as a symptom to reading it as a signal, then into practices that help us metabolise it across body, mind, and spirit. We begin in the individual body, then look outward—to seasons, soil, sunlight, and the structures that surround us. We ask what it means to live cyclically in a linear world, to choose softness in an age that rewards hardness, to find healing not in flight but in rooted presence.

Why the urgency now? Because the breaking point is upon us. Chronic stress has become so normalised that true rest feels strange to many—more threatening than the familiar churn of anxiety or numbness. This is not normal. Nor is it fate.

What if stress is the soul's rebellion against a half-lived life? What if burnout marks not collapse, but a threshold? What if exhaustion is less a flaw than a quiet intelligence, asking to be heard?

Here lies the heart of *Healing Beyond Pills*: the recognition that you are not broken, that your body is not betraying you, that stress may be your ally, speaking only too loudly to ignore. You are not here to be optimised or sedated. You are here to live—wholly, cyclically, with integrity.

This is for those who wish to slow down, not as indulgence but as remembering. For those who know, somewhere beneath the din, that the truest medicine has always been near: in breath, in soil, in the deep silence that follows a question asked with sincerity.

Welcome. Step gently. And let us begin.

Chapter 1
The Noise Beneath the Silence: What Stress Is Really Saying

Stress may be the most examined, commodified, and yet misread phenomenon of our age. We drape it over ourselves like a habitual garment—numbing it with medication, parceling it into therapy sessions, excusing it as the unavoidable tax on achievement. It is framed as a defect, a departure from our supposed baseline of wellness. But perhaps we have mistaken its purpose. What if stress is not the body's stumble into error, but a clear and deliberate signal—encoded in muscle tightness, exhaustion, emotional distance? Not a system collapsing, but a system communicating?

The dominant medical lens tends to treat stress as a malfunctioning reflex—a hyperactive response to external demands. And so the remedies follow suit: dampen the symptoms, restore equilibrium, press on. Yet this approach overlooks the startling intelligence behind the phenomenon. Chronic stress is not simply the wear-and-tear of busy lives; it is the fluent protest of the body on behalf of biological, social, and even spiritual systems that have slipped out of alignment. It is an insistence that our way of living no longer matches our design.

Here, we begin with a reframe: stress is no error. It is a messenger—an evolutionary feedback loop woven from our physiology, cultural conditioning, psychological narratives, and spiritual sensibilities. Its persistence is not evidence of bodily failure, but of a refusal to fall silent.

To hear what it says, we must trade symptom-chasing for systems thinking. Chronic stress does not distribute itself randomly. It shadows inequity, alienation from the natural world, spiritual dislocation, the thinning of community bonds. It flourishes where productivity is prized above presence, perfection above authenticity, consumption above connection. When our surroundings contradict our most fundamental needs—security, rhythm, belonging—the nervous system does not merely adapt. It resists. That resistance often shows up as relentless activation, collapse, or a drifting away from one's own sensations.

None of this is to romanticise stress or downplay its corrosive potential. Left unchecked, it is implicated in a host of chronic diseases, from cardiac disorders to autoimmune breakdowns. But its persistence tells a coherent story: one of unresolved trauma, of values lived out of sync, of emotions locked away, and of cultural frameworks that reward the very conditions that breed distress. Seen in its entirety, the stress response is not just a reflex—it is a compass, one we have been stubbornly ignoring.

Enter polyvagal theory, Dr Stephen Porges's contribution to our understanding of the autonomic nervous system. This model moves us beyond the old binary of 'fight-or-flight' versus 'rest-and-digest'. Instead, it reveals a layered, adaptive system engaged in constant surveillance for cues of safety or danger—a process he terms neuroception. When safety registers, we become expansive, engaged, creative. When threat—however faint—is sensed, the body narrows its scope, prioritising immediate survival at the cost of long-term vitality.

It's why two people in identical circumstances can react in utterly different ways. A routine meeting for one may trigger alarm for another. Such responses are not conscious choices, but the outcome of deep, non-verbal memory—shaped by upbringing, social imprinting, even inherited wounds. Understood this way, stress is neither irrational nor weak. It is, in fact, exquisitely contextual.

Healing, then, is not a matter of simply unwinding on cue or thinking more positively. It is about re-tuning our neurobiological relationship with the world—a shift that cannot be achieved in the intellect alone. It requires experiences that rebuild a sense of safety, both within the skin and within the fabric of life.

But safety is a rare currency in a culture that rewards speed over stillness, noise over quiet, independence over interdependence. Our very infrastructure conspires to sustain a stress state—pinging phones, snarled commutes, precarious employment, fractured attention. These are not isolated irritants; they are ongoing disruptions to the rhythms our bodies rely on, keeping us in a subtle but constant state of activation until we burn out in body and in spirit.

Here, psychology meets mythology in the idea of soul-loss. Clinically, it may be described as dissociation—a self-protective uncoupling from experience that overwhelms. In shamanic terms, it is the splintering of vital essence after trauma or prolonged hardship. However one names it, the pattern is the same: under sustained overwhelm, the self begins to withdraw.

In this state, life turns mechanical. The colour drains from experience. People may function at work, maintain relationships, but feel hollow at the core. This is not mere fatigue or garden-variety sadness; it is a profound estrangement from self and meaning. Modern burnout often hides here—not simply in overwork, but in underconnection to what matters. We become streamlined but empty, driven yet inert.

This brings us to the least recognised of stress responses: freeze. Unlike fight or flight, freeze—immobilisation, dorsal vagal shutdown—is the body's last-ditch survival move when escape or confrontation is impossible. It manifests as numbness, disconnection, emotional dullness, a kind of internal folding-in. Many living with long-term stress are not buzzing with anxiety but moving through life as if under glass.

Freeze is not weakness. It is a shield. Yet when sustained, it can teach the body to live as if safety is never guaranteed. The world becomes a terrain of quiet threat. People function—sometimes impressively—but without the freedom to feel. And because freeze looks less dramatic than panic or rage, it slips under the radar of conventional medicine. You'll find it in the fatigued CEO, the autopilot caregiver, the student quietly drowning in obligations.

Western medicine, intent on isolating causes and prescribing fixes, treats the symptoms—high blood pressure, digestive distress, sleeplessness—while often missing the larger question: why is the body still sounding the alarm?

To answer, we must learn the body's language. We must pay attention to the quieter messages: the joy that has ebbed without notice, the breath that never quite deepens, the small ache we've written off as habit. Chronic stress is more often the weight of countless ignored signals than the impact of a single blow.

This chapter will walk you through those signals. We will trace how experience is etched into the nervous system, how beliefs sculpt biology, how the language of soul-loss can illuminate modern disconnection. We will explore the freeze state not only as physiology, but as a filter shaping perception itself. And we will examine how cultural myths frame stress as fragility or moral failure—when in truth it is neither.

You will not emerge from these pages with stress 'solved'. But you will see it differently. You will begin to recognise that stress is not asking you to soldier on, optimise your routine, or sit more often in lotus pose. It is asking you to listen—with the body, the breath, the memories, the instincts.

Stress is not random. It is relational. It is the body's insistence on telling the truth, long after the rest of us have learned to keep quiet. The language is still there, waiting. We need only remember how to hear it.

Stress as a Messenger, Not a Malfunction

Stress, as we have been taught to understand it, is something to be reduced, managed, or avoided—an unwanted residue of modern life, corrosive to health and performance. It is treated, culturally and medically, as if it were a fault in the system: a biochemical misfire, a cognitive failure, a temporary lapse in personal resilience. But this framing is intellectually shallow and clinically insufficient. Stress is not a malfunction. It is a message. And until we decode its language rather than suppress its symptoms, we will continue to misread the body's most sophisticated signals.

To reframe stress as a messenger is to return to its evolutionary purpose. Human physiology has not fallen behind the times. The autonomic nervous system is not broken. On the contrary, it is highly responsive and exquisitely tuned to our interpretations of the world. Stress, in its acute form, is a life-preserving mechanism—an ancient signal that once mobilised our ancestors to flee predators, survive hunger, or navigate volatile tribal politics. It is not the response itself that has become maladaptive, but the chronic conditions under which it is now activated. We have created environments that trigger emergency states without resolution, vigilance without reprieve, and effort without restoration.

What we call chronic stress is not the body misbehaving—it is the body speaking clearly about a deeper incongruence. It is not merely biochemical; it is contextual, relational, and existential. The rising incidence of burnout, anxiety disorders, and autoimmune illnesses reflects not individual failure, but systemic dissonance. We are living in ways that contradict what our biology recognises as safe, meaningful, and coherent. Stress, in this light, becomes a mirror—not of weakness, but of wisdom.

Consider the disjunction between the pace of contemporary life and the tempo of human physiology. The body evolved over millennia in rhythm with the sun, the seasons, and the cycles of exertion and rest. Today, it is subjected to non-stop input: artificial lighting, digital noise, social fragmentation, economic precarity. We expect the nervous system to adapt, and in many ways, it does. But adaptation does not mean health. It means compensation. And the cost of that compensation—when the sympathetic system is persistently activated, and the parasympathetic response is chronically inhibited—is cumulative dysfunction: disrupted sleep, impaired digestion, hormonal imbalances, and neuroinflammatory states. These are not bugs in the system. They are intelligible signals that the organism is operating outside its tolerable limits.

The reductionist language of stress as a "disorder" or "imbalance" strips it of meaning. When we pathologise stress, we fail to ask what it is pointing toward. We intervene in the noise without tracing its source. The body becomes something to silence, the symptoms something to medicate, and the mind something to manage. But what if the anxiety isn't irrational? What if the exhaustion is not a sign of laziness but of cumulative overextension? What if the burnout is a refusal—by the body and the psyche—to continue performing a version of life that no longer makes sense?

Stress, when chronic, is not an uninvited guest. It is a signal of misalignment between internal needs and external demands. This misalignment may occur at any level—physical, emotional, relational, existential. The professional forced to operate in a value-conflicted corporate structure, the caregiver navigating invisible labour without support, the student submerged in performance anxiety without authentic meaning—each is experiencing stress not as failure but as feedback. The body is not just tired. It is trying to say *no* in a culture that only values *yes*.

The nervous system, especially through the lens of polyvagal theory, is a storyteller. It narrates our lived experience not in words, but in patterns of activation, regulation, and shutdown. When we encounter threat, the sympathetic branch activates—heart rate increases, muscles tense, senses sharpen. If the threat is resolved, the parasympathetic system restores balance. But when safety is not restored, or when threat is sustained over time—through micro-aggressions, economic instability, unresolved trauma—the body does not return to baseline. Instead, it enters a defensive posture, subtly or overtly, that becomes habitual. Over time, these patterns embed themselves into posture, digestion, attention span, sleep cycles, even personality.

And here lies one of the most overlooked truths in stress research: the body doesn't simply react to what is objectively happening. It responds to what it *perceives*—and those perceptions are shaped by memory, meaning, belief, and culture. Two people may walk into the same room and experience radically different physiological responses. One may feel energised and open; the other may feel under threat. This is not irrationality. It is neuroception—the body's way of scanning for cues of safety or danger, beneath conscious awareness.

This means that stress is not merely about workload or noise levels or deadlines. It is also about narratives. The internal stories we carry—about worth, belonging, competence, danger—directly influence how the nervous system calibrates its responses. If one grew up in an environment where rest was punished or vulnerability equated with danger, even positive experiences may trigger stress. Healing, therefore, is not only about behavioural change. It is about re-educating the nervous system to perceive safety where it once saw threat, and to reclaim connection where it once retreated into isolation.

And yet, most interventions for stress do not address this deeper layer. They offer coping mechanisms but neglect meaning. They offer strategies but ignore story. The standard prescription for stress—time off work, cognitive-behavioural techniques, perhaps a mindfulness app—may offer temporary relief, but often fail to address why the stress emerged in the first place. Without this depth, we risk treating stress like noise pollution, rather than decoding it as a sophisticated internal warning system.

To do so, we must look not only inward, but also outward. Chronic stress is not merely personal. It is political. It is ecological. It is cultural. We are living in systems that make sustained wellbeing nearly impossible for many. Economic models that commodify attention and incentivise overwork; educational institutions that reward conformity over creativity; healthcare systems that medicate symptoms while ignoring root causes—all of these contribute to a landscape in which chronic stress is not an individual failure, but a predictable outcome.

Reframing stress as a messenger shifts the moral lens as well. It removes blame. It invites inquiry. It allows us to ask: What is being asked of me that contradicts my deeper values? What part of me has been silenced in the name of success? What rhythm has my body been calling for, and how long have I ignored it?

This is not about becoming stress-free—a fantasy that serves neither science nor soul. It is about becoming stress-literate. It is about recognising that stress is information. And like all information, its usefulness depends on how we interpret it. Some stress is unavoidable, even essential—it signals growth, change, the need for boundaries. But chronic, unresolved stress is different. It is not an unfortunate by-product of a fast-paced life. It is a plea for recalibration.

To truly engage with stress as a messenger requires humility. It requires that we stop assuming we know what is best for the body and instead listen to what it is trying to tell us. This listening is not passive. It requires discernment, inquiry, and often courage. Because sometimes the message is that we need to stop doing what everyone else is doing. That we need to leave environments that reward self-betrayal. That we need to rest, not as a luxury, but as an act of defiance against a system that benefits from our depletion.

The shift from seeing stress as a malfunction to seeing it as a message is not merely semantic. It changes how we relate to ourselves. It reclaims the body as an intelligent, responsive system rather than a fragile machine. It reframes symptoms as signals rather than flaws. And it reminds us that resilience is not the ability to endure more, but the ability to respond more wisely.

This chapter, and this book, do not aim to eliminate stress. They aim to illuminate it. To understand its origins, its expressions, and its implications. Not to silence the alarm, but to finally answer the call. Because beneath the noise, stress is saying something. And what it's saying, often, is: *this is not sustainable. This is not aligned. This is not true to who you are.*

That message is not one to fear. It is one to heed. And in doing so, we do not move further into fragility—we move toward coherence, toward wholeness, and toward a form of health that honours not only the body's needs, but its profound intelligence.

Biology Meets Belief: How Our Nervous System Interprets the World

The body is not simply a machine responding to objective stimuli; it is a living archive of experiences, expectations, and inherited meanings. When it comes to stress and safety, the nervous system doesn't wait for conscious analysis. It scans, sorts, and responds in real time—faster than thought, deeper than language. This scanning process, known as *neuroception*, determines whether we engage, retreat, fight, freeze, or shut down. And it does so based not just on present circumstances, but on what our biology *believes* about the world. These beliefs—shaped by memory, trauma, culture, and story—are encoded as patterns of perception. Understanding stress, therefore, requires more than biological metrics. It requires a reckoning with how belief shapes biology.

At the heart of this discussion is the polyvagal theory, a groundbreaking model developed by neuroscientist Dr Stephen Porges. It dismantles the simplistic binary of fight-or-flight versus rest-and-digest, offering instead a nuanced map of the autonomic nervous system. According to this theory, we navigate life through a three-tiered hierarchy of responses, each governed by a different branch of the vagus nerve. The most evolutionarily recent is the *ventral vagal complex*, which supports social engagement, calm states, and feelings of safety. When we feel secure, connected, and seen, this system dominates. Our breath slows, our facial muscles soften, our voice steadies, and we become capable of empathy, creativity, and relational depth.

When safety is compromised, the system downshifts. The *sympathetic branch* takes over, mobilising the body for action—racing heart, dilated pupils, tightened muscles. This state is designed for short bursts of exertion, not sustained living. If the threat persists or becomes overwhelming, the body defaults to the oldest evolutionary defence: *dorsal vagal shutdown*. In this state, energy collapses. Emotion numbs. Disconnection replaces urgency. Many people living with chronic stress oscillate between the agitation of sympathetic arousal and the numb withdrawal of dorsal shutdown—often without knowing why. Their nervous system is not malfunctioning; it is responding exactly as designed, based on its reading of the world.

What determines that reading is not just present conditions, but the internal narrative of the self in relation to the world. If a person was raised in an environment where expression led to punishment, or where affection was inconsistent, the nervous system may interpret intimacy not as safety, but as risk. Similarly, someone who experienced early chaos may interpret routine as stifling, even threatening. These interpretations live in the body—not as abstract thoughts, but as embodied truths. The nervous system does not distinguish between *real* threat and *perceived* threat. It only responds to whether it feels safe. And feeling safe is often less about what is happening, and more about what has happened before.

This is where biology meets belief. Our body's response to stress is shaped by past experience, but also by the stories we tell ourselves about what those experiences mean. The nervous system listens closely to these narratives. A woman who has internalised that she must perform perfectly to be loved may experience minor critique as a life-threatening event—not because she lacks perspective, but because her nervous system has equated failure with abandonment. A man taught that vulnerability is weakness may feel anxious not in moments of danger, but in moments of emotional intimacy. Their stress responses are not irrational—they are contextual. They reflect a nervous system that has calibrated itself to survive particular realities, and continues to interpret the world through that lens.

This lens is not formed in isolation. It is shaped by culture, family systems, generational trauma, and collective myth. Our ancestors did not use the language of neurobiology, but they encoded nervous system intelligence in story. Myths across cultures describe beings who retreat into caves when overwhelmed, who lose their voices when betrayed, who freeze in the face of injustice. These are not just moral tales; they are somatic metaphors. The archetype of the wounded hero, the silent child, the rageful outcast—each reflects a nervous system pattern, dressed in narrative clothing. To dismiss these as mere fiction is to underestimate the role of collective storytelling in shaping our embodied responses.

Modern neuroscience is, in a sense, catching up to what traditional cultures encoded through symbolism. The nervous system speaks a language older than reason. It does not respond to logic, but to *felt* meaning. A patient may intellectually understand that a dog is not dangerous, yet experience full-body panic at the sight of one. This is not irrational—it is the nervous system honouring a narrative written in the body. To heal from chronic stress, then, is not simply to regulate the nervous system through breathwork or diet. It is to excavate these embodied narratives, to understand which beliefs the body has mistaken for truth, and to create new experiences that rewire perception at its root.

Real-world applications of this insight are profound. In psychotherapy, somatic approaches such as Sensorimotor Psychotherapy and Somatic Experiencing do not simply ask "What happened to you?"—they ask "What did your body learn from what happened?" and "What does your body still believe to be true?" In trauma-informed coaching, practitioners track subtle cues—voice tone, micro-movements, eye gaze—not as indicators of pathology, but as expressions of neurophysiological state. Even in organisational leadership, polyvagal principles are being applied to reshape how meetings are conducted, how conflict is mediated, and how psychological safety is cultivated.

The implications extend into education, criminal justice, parenting, and spiritual practice. A teacher who understands that a student's defiance may reflect sympathetic activation rather than insolence can respond with regulation rather than punishment. A parent who sees their child's withdrawal not as disobedience but as dorsal shutdown can offer presence instead of pressure. A spiritual guide who recognises that a seeker's inability to meditate may stem not from laziness but from an over-activated nervous system can tailor practices accordingly. These are not just clinical insights. They are cultural imperatives.

But insight alone is not sufficient. Polyvagal-informed understanding must be translated into embodied change. This requires more than mindfulness. It requires *mindsight*—a term coined by Dr Daniel Siegel to describe the capacity to sense and shape our internal states with curiosity and compassion. Mindsight is not a mental trick; it is a discipline of attention that builds nervous system fluency over time. It allows us to notice when we are slipping into activation or shutdown, and to intervene not through willpower, but through relationship—to breath, to body, to others, and to story.

Belief is not just psychological. It is biological. Every belief carries a posture, a breath pattern, a neurochemical signature. When we say we feel "safe," we are describing a physiological reality: vagal tone, heart-rate variability, oxytocin levels, muscle relaxation. Safety is not a concept. It is a state. And because it is a state, it can be cultivated—not only through external security, but through internal coherence. The more often we return to states of safety, the more the nervous system begins to expect it. Over time, safety becomes not just an experience, but a belief. And that belief, once embedded in the body, becomes a new baseline for interpreting the world.

This reorientation has profound ethical implications. It means we cannot assume what others are experiencing based on what appears rational. It requires a shift from judgement to curiosity, from diagnosis to dialogue. When someone reacts "out of proportion," they are not failing—they are expressing. When someone cannot "just calm down," they are not resisting—they are surviving. To be trauma-informed is not merely to know the research. It is to live as if nervous systems are always in the room, always listening, always responding. It is to ask not only "What is wrong with you?" but "What has shaped the way your body perceives this moment?"

Ultimately, the polyvagal lens restores dignity to the stress response. It reveals the nervous system not as a broken circuit, but as an adaptive storyteller—one that learns from the past, interprets the present, and shapes the future through its beliefs. To change the story, we must first hear it. And to hear it, we must stop demanding rationality from a system that evolved to prioritise survival.

This is not a retreat from science into sentimentality. On the contrary, it is science at its most humane—recognising that data lives not only in charts and scans, but in the lived realities of breath, heart, and gut. By bridging neuroscience with narrative, biology with belief, we gain not only a richer understanding of stress but a deeper respect for the intelligence of the body. And it is from that respect—not control, not suppression—that real healing begins.

When the Soul Goes Offline

There are moments in modern life when a person walks into a room and no one truly arrives. The body enters, gestures are made, words are spoken, but something essential is missing—an interior aliveness, a sense of presence. Increasingly, this state of internal absence has become both common and accepted. It is not dramatic enough to raise alarm, nor visibly dysfunctional enough to warrant diagnosis. Yet it defines the lived experience of many navigating contemporary existence: going through motions, performing tasks, achieving goals, all while feeling hollowed out at the core. What's gone missing is not capacity, but contact—with one's own emotional depth, vitality, and coherence. This is not simply exhaustion. It is something more profound. In both psychology and ancestral traditions, there is language for this phenomenon. Psychology calls it *dissociation*. Indigenous medicine names it *soul-loss*.

To speak of the soul in a clinical or academic context often elicits discomfort. The word resists quantification, does not sit neatly in diagnostic manuals, and invites interpretations that vary across culture, religion, and worldview. Yet across disciplines, the reality it points to—a severing of the self from its own fullness—is undeniable. In psychological terms, dissociation is the mind's way of coping with overwhelming experience. It is an adaptive, protective mechanism. When pain is too great or circumstances too unstable, the psyche distances itself from the present in order to survive. This may involve depersonalisation, emotional numbing, memory fragmentation, or a vague sense of being "not really here." What begins as a survival strategy can, over time, become a default mode—especially in environments that continually reinforce stress and suppress integration.

In shamanic and indigenous frameworks, the idea of soul-loss offers a parallel but more relational understanding. It describes not only a psychological phenomenon, but an energetic dislocation—a part of the person's essence that flees or disconnects in the face of trauma, grief, or prolonged misalignment. This soul-fragment is not considered destroyed but displaced, living elsewhere until conditions are safe enough to return. Traditional healers do not treat soul-loss with talk therapy or pharmaceuticals. They engage in ritual, ceremony, and intentional acts of witnessing designed to create the right conditions for return. The language is spiritual, but the implications are strikingly somatic: wholeness is not achieved by controlling the mind, but by restoring relationship with lost parts of the self.

These two lenses—psychological dissociation and shamanic soul-loss—may seem conceptually different, but they converge on a shared truth: *the self can become estranged from itself.* Whether described as neurophysiological disintegration or spiritual fragmentation, the experience is viscerally real. Individuals report feeling cut off from their emotions, unable to feel joy, unable to cry, even when their external lives remain intact. Creativity evaporates. Purpose becomes abstract. Relationships lose their depth. The person continues functioning—meeting deadlines, maintaining appearances—but no longer experiences themselves as fully alive.

Burnout is often the modern expression of this state. Commonly framed as a depletion of energy, burnout is more accurately a depletion of *inner access*. The body keeps going, the calendar stays full, but the interior world becomes thin. There is a flattening of affect, a loss of nuance in perception, a chronic dullness that no amount of rest, supplements, or self-care routines can fully resolve. This is not mere fatigue. It is estrangement. The soul, in metaphorical terms, has gone offline.

Understanding this requires recognising the kinds of environments that produce soul-disconnection. These are often environments that demand high output and low introspection; that reward appearance over authenticity; that punish vulnerability and pathologise emotion. In such contexts, individuals learn to suppress their intuitive signals, override bodily wisdom, and silence inner dissent in order to conform. The nervous system, sensing that true expression is unsafe, gradually narrows the range of felt experience. Over time, this protective narrowing becomes a baseline, and the person forgets what it felt like to be fully connected. It is not a single trauma that causes this disconnection, but a sustained absence of resonance—a life structured in such a way that the soul has no room to speak.

What makes soul-loss particularly insidious is that it often escapes conventional mental health screening. A person may score within normal ranges on anxiety and depression scales, yet report a haunting emptiness—a sense that something is missing but cannot be named. They may feel emotionally detached from their own memories, struggle to access desires, or experience time as compressed and meaningless. This is not simply the result of chemical imbalance. It is the outcome of prolonged disconnection from one's own depth.

Modern neuroscience has begun to catch up with these more ancient insights. Studies on trauma and chronic stress have shown that key brain regions—such as the prefrontal cortex, amygdala, and insular cortex—can undergo measurable changes under conditions of repeated overwhelm or neglect. These changes impact emotional regulation, memory integration, and self-awareness. When viewed through a neurobiological lens, soul-loss is not an esoteric idea, but a measurable shift in how the brain processes identity and connection. The metaphors of ancestral medicine and the metrics of contemporary science are not at odds; they are describing the same phenomenon in different dialects.

The implications for healing are significant. Approaches that rely solely on cognition—rational insight, behavioural change, even verbal expression—are often insufficient for those experiencing soul-disconnection. The path back is not through information alone, but through re-embodiment. Practices such as somatic therapy, expressive arts, ritual, and non-linear movement are increasingly being recognised as essential tools for re-establishing contact with lost aspects of the self. These practices bypass the analytical mind and invite direct sensory, emotional, and symbolic engagement.

In many traditional cultures, healing begins not with diagnosis, but with *witnessing*. The community holds space for the individual not to perform, not to fix, but to be seen. The act of being genuinely seen—by others, by oneself, by the forces one considers sacred—has extraordinary restorative power. It signals to the nervous system that it is once again safe to show up, to feel, to remember. Healing from soul-loss, then, is not a technical fix. It is a re-invitation.

Of course, not all experiences of dissociation are pathological. The ability to temporarily detach from sensation or emotion can be useful—even necessary—in certain circumstances. The problem arises when dissociation becomes chronic, unexamined, and embedded in one's identity. A soldier returning from combat, a survivor of early childhood trauma, a professional in a high-pressure environment—all may develop dissociative habits that initially serve them, but later cost them access to joy, intimacy, and meaning. The challenge is not to eliminate dissociation, but to develop the discernment to know when it is happening, why it is happening, and how to safely return from it.

There is also a larger ethical and cultural dimension to this discussion. We live in a time that increasingly pathologises disconnection while simultaneously designing systems that produce it. Institutions that value standardisation over humanity, technologies that accelerate attention fragmentation, economies that monetise burnout—these are not neutral backdrops. They are active participants in the story of soul-loss. To address dissociation without critiquing the structures that reinforce it is to treat symptoms in isolation. Healing, in this context, must be both personal and political.

Yet the goal is not to recover some idealised state of permanent presence. The soul, like the body, ebbs and flows. There will be moments of departure and return, contraction and expansion. What matters is not whether we are always "online," but whether we notice when we are not—and whether we have the tools, the relationships, and the permission to come back. Healing is less about fixing what's broken and more about re-establishing right relationship: with the body, with emotion, with memory, with meaning.

The soul does not vanish in times of disconnection. It waits. It waits for conditions of safety, resonance, and respect. It waits for silence deep enough to hear its voice. It waits for us to stop performing and start listening. And when those conditions are met—not through force, but through care—it returns. Not in dramatic revelation, but in subtle shifts: a moment of unprompted laughter, a sudden flush of emotion, a dream that feels oddly alive. These are signs that something within has come back online.

To understand burnout, numbness, and chronic disconnection only as individual dysfunctions is to miss the deeper truth. These states are responses—intelligent, adaptive, and worthy of respect. They are evidence not of brokenness, but of the soul's insistence on integrity. When the soul goes offline, it is not abandoning us. It is asking for us to return to something real. And in honouring that request, we begin not just to heal, but to remember what it means to be whole.

From Fight-or-Flight to Freeze-and-Forget

When we talk about stress, the dominant metaphor is one of urgency: rapid heartbeat, narrowed focus, the impulse to act or escape. The fight-or-flight response has become shorthand for how our bodies react to threat—an elegant, time-tested system designed to ensure survival. But this binary model is incomplete. What happens when the threat cannot be fought or fled? What happens when danger is chronic, when the body's signals are repeatedly ignored, or when powerlessness becomes the norm? The answer, increasingly recognised in psychophysiology but still neglected in mainstream medicine, is the *freeze response*—a state not of arousal, but of withdrawal. And with it comes a silent epidemic: emotional numbing, disembodiment, and the quiet erasure of aliveness.

The autonomic nervous system operates in a hierarchical cascade. At its peak, under conditions of safety, is the ventral vagal system—social engagement, openness, curiosity, and regulation. When threat is detected, we drop into sympathetic activation: mobilisation, protection, adrenaline-fuelled readiness. But if neither fighting nor fleeing is possible, the system defaults to its oldest survival strategy—dorsal vagal shutdown. In this state, the body slows, constricts, and retreats. Emotion flattens. Memory blurs. Awareness narrows. It is a biological folding in, a strategic conservation of energy when external safety cannot be achieved.

This freeze state is not a glitch; it is an evolutionary inheritance. Mammals immobilise in the face of predation not only to feign death but to reduce the perception of pain if death is imminent. Humans retain this capacity—though its expression is often subtle and long-lasting. The problem is that we now encounter threats not from predators, but from unrelenting emotional strain, cultural overexertion, relational violation, and chronic uncertainty. These conditions do not elicit immediate physical danger but instead produce a slow, sustained drain on the nervous system. Over time, the stress response shifts from episodic activation to habituated suppression. What begins as fight-or-flight becomes freeze-and-forget.

In real-world terms, this looks like disengagement. Not dramatic panic, but a quiet sense of dislocation: "I'm here, but I don't feel here." People in this state often report difficulty accessing joy, tears, creativity, or even clear thought. Their daily lives may be functional, even high-achieving, but the internal experience is flatlined. They might describe themselves as burnt out, indifferent, disconnected from their body, or emotionally unavailable. From the outside, they appear stable. Internally, they are in a kind of suspended animation.

Modern medicine rarely recognises this state for what it is. The diagnostic frameworks we rely on are skewed toward visible symptoms—hyperarousal, insomnia, irritability, panic attacks. Freeze, by contrast, is quiet. It doesn't raise red flags in short medical appointments or performance reviews. A patient might present with fatigue, brain fog, or low mood, and receive an antidepressant or stimulant. Yet if the root state is dorsal shutdown, these interventions may miss the mark entirely. At best, they temporarily override the symptoms. At worst, they reinforce the disconnection by silencing the very signals that point to deeper dysregulation.

The standard prescription to "manage stress" typically assumes the presence of excess energy—hence the advice to exercise more, meditate harder, take control. But the freeze response is not characterised by excess; it is defined by depletion. Telling someone in dorsal collapse to "just breathe" or "power through" is not just ineffective—it can be retraumatising. It reinforces the cultural belief that numbness is a personal failure, rather than a physiological expression of unresolved overwhelm.

There is also a deeper issue: when the nervous system becomes habituated to shutdown, the mind adapts accordingly. Emotional suppression becomes a coping mechanism. The body is no longer experienced as a trustworthy source of guidance. This is not simply dissociation; it is *disembodiment.* The person lives increasingly in abstraction—in thoughts, roles, or routines—with little access to sensory or affective reality. They may struggle to detect internal cues such as hunger, fatigue, or boundaries. They may intellectualise emotions rather than feel them. Over time, the link between sensation and meaning becomes frayed, and the body is perceived more as an object to manage than a home to inhabit.

This dynamic plays out in countless settings—clinical, educational, corporate—where people are praised for being "resilient" while privately struggling with apathy or inertia. It plays out in communities where trauma is endemic, but expression is stigmatised. It plays out in children who "behave well" because their nervous systems have adapted to suppress emotion as a strategy for survival. In each case, the absence of distress is mistaken for wellness. But stillness is not always serenity. It is sometimes surrender.

One of the most critical insights from somatic therapy and trauma research is that healing the freeze state requires more than insight. It requires *experience*—specifically, experiences that offer the body new templates for safety, mobilisation, and integration. This often begins not with catharsis but with micro-movements: orienting to the environment, tracking breath without manipulation, making eye contact in a supported context. These interventions may seem inconsequential to the untrained observer. But to a nervous system in shutdown, they are seismic.

It is here that conventional medicine's emphasis on symptom suppression shows its limitations. The medical model excels at crisis intervention, but struggles with complexity that unfolds over time. It treats disconnection as secondary—something to tolerate, medicate, or ignore—rather than as a foundational disruption of relational and physiological integrity. Worse, it often pathologises the patient's attempts to cope. A withdrawn person is labelled as depressed. A disengaged student is considered inattentive. A shutdown employee is seen as unmotivated. Rarely is the question asked: *What does this withdrawal protect against? What threat has not yet passed, or never been acknowledged?*

By contrast, many traditional healing systems—including Ayurveda, Chinese medicine, and indigenous somatic practices—recognise the importance of restoring energy flow through subtle, repetitive engagement with the body. They attend not just to symptom but to stagnation, not just to what is wrong but to what is missing. The aim is not simply to return the person to productivity but to reinstate connection—within themselves, with others, and with the rhythms of the natural world. These traditions, often dismissed as unscientific, may in fact be ahead of the curve in their respect for the body's cyclical wisdom.

The freeze state also has ethical implications. In a society that pathologises slowness and idolises constant output, shutdown is often misread. It is seen as laziness, aloofness, or indifference. But these labels fail to recognise the evolutionary logic at work. A system that has been overwhelmed without relief will, eventually, retreat. Not because it is defective, but because it is choosing survival over collapse. To work with this reality requires more than empathy. It requires fluency in nervous system states—an understanding that activation and withdrawal are not opposites, but stages on a spectrum of safety-seeking.

What becomes clear is that healing from freeze is not about pushing through. It is about learning to listen to what the freeze protects. It is about creating conditions of sufficient safety for the body to reawaken its suppressed impulses—movement, sensation, curiosity, pleasure. This reawakening is gradual and must be respected. Too much stimulation too soon can backfire. The body does not respond to force; it responds to invitation.

Ultimately, the transition from freeze-and-forget to feeling-and-integration is not linear. It is not a heroic ascent. It is a slow thaw, often imperceptible from the outside but deeply transformative within. It may begin with a sigh that feels involuntary, a shift in posture, a tear that arises unbidden. These are not small things. They are signs that the nervous system is testing the waters of safety, that life is beginning to return on its own terms.

To recognise the freeze response as a legitimate survival state is to challenge much of what modern society calls functional. It is to question the glorification of disconnection, the medicalisation of adaptation, and the moral judgment we place on those who no longer have the energy to perform wellness. And it is to remind ourselves that beneath every shutdown is a story—not only of what went wrong, but of what the body did so wisely to keep going. That story deserves not just understanding, but honour. And the person living it deserves more than coping strategies. They deserve the possibility of return.

Chapter 2
The Culture of Collapse: Why We're Wired to Burn Out

There is something unsettling about inhabiting an era in which stillness itself can feel unsafe. The simple acts—pausing, stepping away, allowing oneself to rest—now appear almost illicit, as though idleness might dismantle the machinery of a life engineered for speed. In a culture calibrated for constant acceleration, the human nervous system struggles to keep pace. Worth is mistaken for busyness; identity for output. We are not merely overstimulated anymore—we are structurally overwhelmed. What once appeared as episodic exhaustion has hardened into a steady state of dysregulation. Burnout is no longer the rare collapse at the end of a hard season; it is fast becoming the ambient condition of modern life.

This chapter opens with a claim that will sit uncomfortably with some: burnout is not only tolerated by our culture—it is manufactured. The conditions that create it are not incidental but celebrated, then repackaged into palatable "cures" sold back to us at a profit. A civilisation obsessed with growth, efficiency, and relentless striving cannot make space for genuine balance without betraying its own values. And so it teaches us to burn out discreetly, to internalise fatigue as personal inadequacy, and to seek relief in half-measures that soothe without ever dismantling the cause. In such a context, genuine healing begins to look like quiet rebellion.

At the root of this engineered collapse lies our altered relationship with speed. Over the last century, time itself has been retextured—not in volume, but in feel. The industrial clock once cut labour loose from the sun; the digital age has since diced our attention into units to be harvested. We no longer experience time as a rhythm, but as a commodity—each minute something to be spent, each hour a vessel for measurable output. What this breeds is not simply tiredness, but a peculiar kind of forgetting: a loss of the body's memory for slowness, for integration, for the kind of rest that knits us back together.

This amnesia is cultivated early. Schools that reward achievement over curiosity; workplaces that prize round-the-clock accessibility over discernment. Productivity has drifted from being a measure of work to being a measure of worth. Fatigue signals virtue. Unavailability is suspect. Rest is permissible only when it can be folded into a performance of efficiency. This is no cultural glitch—it is a structure, an economic logic that thrives on depletion.

And here we meet a paradox: the wellness industry, which might appear poised to challenge this disconnection, often serves to reinforce it. What began as a reclamation of bodily wisdom has been subsumed into the same market calculus. Yoga sold as lifestyle branding; mindfulness compressed into app-friendly microdoses; nutrition reframed as optimisation for peak output. Even rest is marketed as a means to return to the grind more effectively. The metric replaces the soul. Wellness becomes another product, peddled to those already hollowed out by the culture that promotes it.

True healing does not occur in such containers. It germinates in spaces immune to commodification—in moments too slow to monetise, too relational for algorithms, too unpolished for corporate rollout. Real healing is rarely pretty. It asks for discomfort, for relinquishing certain ambitions, for unpicking the very values by which we have been measuring ourselves. It is less about adding new practices than subtracting the ones that keep us unwell. It asks not, "What else can I do?" but "What am I willing to stop doing?"

Few concepts reveal this distortion more clearly than "self-care." Once rooted in radical, often collective, traditions of self-preservation against systemic harm, it has been hollowed by consumerism into an aesthetic: candles, skincare regimens, luxury baths. Harmless in themselves, but no substitute for care in the truest sense. Real care is interdependent. It flows in cycles of giving and receiving. It considers not only your needs, but who helps meet them—and how you will, in turn, help to meet theirs.

This is the pivot we must make if burnout is to be understood as cultural, not merely personal. The nervous system, as trauma research reminds us, heals in relationship. It calibrates in the presence of safe others, in environments that move with our rhythms, in stretches of time that are unstructured and unclaimed by productivity. Yet modern life moves us in the opposite direction: towards disconnection, haste, fragmentation. Even leisure is booked into the diary. Even rest is staged.

To reclaim rest, then, is not just to sleep more, but to treat it as an act of defiance—especially for those whose bodies have been historically commodified or surveilled. Think of Tricia Hersey and The Nap Ministry, reframing rest as a refusal to be reduced to labour, as a way of repaying the debts of extraction. Rest, here, is not avoidance; it is repair. A remembering of the body's ancient rhythms in a world that would have us forget.

Older traditions, still anchored to land and season, have always known what we have tried to transcend: rest is not a luxury earned through toil, but an elemental requirement of life. Ritual calendars, agricultural cycles, community observances—they all worked with the alternation of growth and dormancy, activity and stillness. Ignore such cycles, and you do not outwit biology; you rupture it. The resulting fatigue, hormonal chaos, and immune fragility are not breakdowns—they are the body's eloquent protests.

Here, we will go deeper into these themes: how speed warps perception, how the market capture of healing distorts its purpose, why genuine care cannot be sustained without returning to shared rhythms. We will map burnout not through individual choices alone, but through the structures that have normalised our separation from our own bodies. We will strip away the polished language of the wellness economy to recover something older and truer: the lexicon of reciprocity, coherence, and pace.

This is not a denunciation of ambition, but an interrogation of the bargain on which our ambitions rest. Who gains from our perpetual motion? What do our calendars say about our values? Which of our innate rhythms have been overridden, and what would it cost—or restore—to trust them again?

By the time these pages are done, you will not hold a neat solution. But you may carry a sharper lens. You might recognise that the body's pull towards stillness is not idleness—it is intelligence. That the craving for quiet is not fragility—it is memory. That your exhaustion is not a flaw—it is information.

This, then, is the culture of collapse. Not an inevitability, but a symptom of forgetting the wisdom of limits. And to remember, we will have to slow—awkwardly, urgently, now.

Speed as Spiritual Amnesia

There is a particular kind of disorientation that occurs when a person moves too fast for too long. It's not just physical fatigue or mental overload—it's a deeper sense of loss, as though something essential has quietly slipped out of reach. This is not simply about doing too much. It's about forgetting *how* to be. We find ourselves increasingly efficient and yet internally dislocated, fluent in task management but strangers to inner rhythm. The modern obsession with speed, productivity, and constant availability does more than fray the edges of our attention—it erodes the deeper architecture of coherence. In moving faster, we lose our felt sense of time, space, and self. We mistake acceleration for evolution. What gets left behind is not merely rest, but memory: *the memory of how to be human in a way that honours biology, spirit, and relational integrity.*

We are not machines designed to scale indefinitely. Human beings evolved with cycles—circadian, seasonal, emotional, relational. These cycles are not optional embellishments. They are physiological imperatives. The endocrine system, for example, relies on rhythmic secretion of hormones to maintain homeostasis. Cortisol peaks in the morning, melatonin at night. The digestive system functions optimally when given predictable intervals. Even cognitive performance waxes and wanes in natural ultradian rhythms, typically every 90 to 120 minutes. But contemporary life is structured in ways that deliberately override these rhythms. We flatten the variability, compress the pauses, and fill every pocket of time with output. The result is not increased efficiency, but chronic dysregulation.

This dysregulation is cumulative and systemic. The body learns to adapt to perpetual stimulation, but at a cost. Sympathetic dominance—marked by heightened cortisol, elevated heart rate, and suppressed digestion—becomes the baseline. People lose access to parasympathetic states, where repair, integration, and connection occur. Over time, this produces not just burnout, but a kind of somatic amnesia. The body forgets how to downshift. Stillness becomes unfamiliar, even intolerable. Attempts to rest are met not with relief, but with anxiety or guilt. The person may lie in bed unable to sleep, or take a day off only to compulsively check emails. The problem is not just external pressure—it's internal pacing that no longer responds to the cues of the body, but to the demands of a culture addicted to speed.

The language of productivity has seeped so deeply into identity that it now shapes how people evaluate their worth. Phrases like "I was so productive today" have become stand-ins for "I mattered today." Time is no longer experienced as cyclical or relational but as linear and extractive. Every minute must be optimised, every hour accounted for. This instrumentalisation of time mirrors industrial and economic logics that value scale over depth. The factory model of labour—originally applied to external production—has been internalised. Now we produce ourselves: better, faster, more. Leisure, when it happens, is often performative. Even so-called rest is monetised, stylised, and marketed back to us as a lifestyle brand.

This has profound implications for the nervous system, which does not recognise brand strategy but responds to lived rhythm. When we abandon natural tempos, we lose coherence between body and context. This lack of coherence is felt as anxiety, fatigue, brain fog, disconnection, and chronic inflammation. Yet instead of treating the root disruption, the dominant response is to mask the symptoms—through caffeine, stimulants, productivity hacks, and surface-level wellness practices. Meditation becomes another box to tick. Breathwork is squeezed between meetings. We attempt to *perform* regulation without ever engaging the deeper architecture of safety and rest.

Critically, this disruption of rhythm is not experienced equally across populations. Those living in marginalised bodies—Black, Indigenous, disabled, immigrant, queer—are often forced to navigate multiple temporalities at once: the pressured pace of dominant economic systems and the subtle, often invisible rhythms of intergenerational trauma and vigilance. The nervous system under systemic threat cannot afford to slow down. The cost of rest is higher when safety is not guaranteed. Thus, the call to reclaim rhythm is not a universal luxury—it is a context-dependent necessity. Any conversation about rest and slowness must be intersectional, or it risks replicating the same injustices it seeks to repair.

There is also a spiritual cost to living at unsustainable speeds. Not necessarily in a religious sense, but in the existential one. The part of us that orients toward meaning—toward beauty, connection, transcendence—requires spaciousness. It cannot be hurried. Reflection, grief, wonder, and awe all require a kind of slowness that modern life often denies. The constant noise of urgency leaves little room for insight to emerge. Silence becomes threatening. Pauses feel like inefficiency. In this state, people lose not only their sense of peace but their ability to *sense*, full stop. The subtle intuition that guides right action, that nourishes relationships, that keeps people tethered to values—it dulls under pressure.

Spiritual amnesia, then, is not forgetting doctrine. It is forgetting how to access the conditions in which realisation occurs. It is not a failure of belief but a failure of tempo. It is the inability to align inner life with outer rhythm. And it leads not just to fatigue, but to confusion. People begin to ask questions like "Why do I feel so numb?" or "Why does everything feel like too much and not enough at the same time?" These are not just emotional issues—they are temporal. They are the signs of a nervous system and a psyche that have lost access to natural pacing.

Recovering internal rhythm requires more than scheduling time off. It requires dismantling the internalised logic that says rest must be earned. It means creating lives structured around integration, not interruption. For some, this might involve reinstating meal rituals, tech-free evenings, or boundaries around work hours. For others, it may mean reconnecting with ancestral practices that embedded rhythm into daily life: prayer, music, communal gatherings, observing lunar or agricultural cycles. These are not quaint traditions. They are technologies of coherence.

This reorientation must also happen collectively. Individual efforts to slow down are often unsustainable without cultural reinforcement. A person cannot heal nervous system dysregulation while embedded in a work culture that pathologises rest or a family system that equates stillness with laziness. Communities need to reclaim shared rhythms—weekly pauses, communal rituals, protected time for non-productive presence. This is not nostalgia. It is infrastructure. Without it, healing becomes an isolated, uphill battle.

The broader challenge is this: to build cultures that do not equate acceleration with advancement. To remember that speed, while useful in moments, is not a stable organising principle for life. There is no innovation that can replace the human need for rhythm, no app that can automate repair, no shortcut to integration. The body cannot be optimised indefinitely. The spirit cannot be ignored without consequence.

What we call burnout is often the final signal of a long-standing temporal mismatch between the body's needs and the culture's expectations. It is not a crisis of stamina but of tempo. It is not a lack of resilience but a result of living too far outside the bounds of what the human nervous system can sustain. To heal, we must remember. And to remember, we must slow down—not just as individuals, but as communities, as institutions, as species.

Slowness is not in opposition to progress. It is its precondition. Without rhythm, there is no sustainable creativity, no embodied leadership, no real relationship. Reclaiming slowness is not retreating from life—it is returning to it on terms that honour the body, the earth, and the parts of ourselves we have forgotten in our pursuit of more. To do this is not easy. But it is essential. Because speed may help us get ahead—but it will not help us come home.

Healing in a World That Profits from Sickness

One of the least examined yet most consequential realities of modern healthcare is that it operates within an economic system that does not benefit from people becoming well. Illness, not health, is profitable. Chronic conditions, not resolution, drive sustained revenue. What we often call "healthcare" is in fact a sprawling sickness management industry—highly technical, fiercely competitive, and increasingly commercialised. This is not a critique of medical science or of the many skilled professionals who work within the system with integrity. It is a reckoning with the structures that govern what counts as treatment, what is reimbursed, what is studied, and—perhaps most insidiously—what is ignored.

At the heart of this problem lies commodification. Healing, in its most authentic form, is slow, relational, and often incompatible with standardisation. But capitalism does not reward slowness. It rewards scalability. And so healing is rebranded, repackaged, and reinserted into the market as product, protocol, or platform. Wellness becomes a line of supplements, a lab-generated smoothie, a five-step detox plan. Yoga, once a spiritual discipline, is remade into branded boutique classes. Meditation is distilled into mindfulness apps with daily streaks and push notifications. Even trauma therapy is now sold through algorithmically optimised self-help content promising transformation in 30 days. The more personal the ailment, the more profitable the solution. The more chronic the condition, the more consistent the revenue.

To fully understand why authentic healing is so often marginalised, we must examine the economics of the system. In most industrialised countries, particularly those with privatised or insurance-based models, healthcare is a volume-based business. Reimbursement is tied to procedures, not outcomes. Pharmaceutical companies are incentivised to develop treatments that require lifelong adherence rather than those that resolve root causes. Hospitals and clinics are financially rewarded for high throughput, not for relational depth. Preventative care, when it is offered, is often narrowly defined—screenings and metrics, not structural interventions or social determinants of health.

This systemic bias distorts the medical gaze. Conditions that can be tracked with biomarkers, diagnosed with clear criteria, and treated with patented medications rise to the top of funding and research priorities. Meanwhile, illnesses that require nuanced understanding—complex trauma, chronic fatigue, fibromyalgia, long COVID, autoimmune dysregulation—are often dismissed or psychologised. Their ambiguity makes them hard to monetise. The result is a widespread pattern of patients being disbelieved, gaslit, or routed through endless referrals, each yielding little more than symptom management.

This institutional blind spot is particularly visible in the treatment of chronic stress. Though now recognised as a leading contributor to everything from cardiovascular disease to immune dysfunction, chronic stress is rarely addressed at its roots. The dominant approach involves either pharmacological intervention—SSRIs, anxiolytics, beta-blockers—or superficial behavioural prescriptions: exercise more, practise mindfulness, get better sleep. These recommendations are not wrong, but they are incomplete. They treat stress as an individual issue divorced from context. What is left out is the social, economic, and cultural machinery that generates and perpetuates stress as a structural condition. The single mother working two jobs without childcare. The gig worker with no healthcare benefits. The migrant labourer facing systemic discrimination. For them, stress is not a "lifestyle issue"—it is a predictable outcome of the systems they inhabit.

Mainstream medicine is structurally ill-equipped to engage with this level of complexity. It fragments the human experience into organ systems and diagnostic codes. It privileges symptom over story. And it separates the body from the society that shapes it. As a result, many people turn to alternative or traditional forms of healing—not necessarily because these are more effective, but because they are more relational, more contextual, and more respectful of the individual's lived experience. In many cases, people feel *seen* for the first time—not as cases to be solved, but as human beings to be heard.

This is not to romanticise alternative medicine, which has its own issues of quality control, overpromising, and commodification. But it does highlight something that mainstream models consistently miss: *healing is not merely the absence of symptoms—it is the restoration of coherence between the self and the world.* And coherence cannot be standardised. It requires time, trust, and attunement—all things that the market devalues. In this sense, true healing is subversive. It resists reduction. It demands space for complexity.

Real-world examples make this tension painfully clear. Consider the rise of "functional medicine" and "integrative health," which promise a more holistic approach to care. In principle, these fields aim to look at the whole person, not just the disease. In practice, many such clinics cater to the affluent, offering personalised protocols that are financially out of reach for most people. Similarly, psychedelic therapy—once the province of indigenous ritual and community-based healing—is now being rapidly commercialised, with venture capitalists investing heavily in clinics, patents, and proprietary treatment models. Even the language of trauma, once grounded in social justice and collective recovery, is now frequently deployed in marketing copy for luxury wellness brands.

This commercial drift leads to a form of what anthropologist Joseph Dumit called *"objective self-fashioning"*—the endless optimisation of the self according to medical and technological standards. It creates consumers who are perpetually in need of tuning, testing, and tweaking. Under the guise of health, we are encouraged to outsource our intuition, to trust biometric feedback over felt experience, to conflate compliance with wellness. The result is a subtle erosion of self-trust. The person becomes a project. And healing becomes a lifelong purchase.

But outside these models, another story is unfolding. In community clinics, grassroots mutual aid networks, indigenous collectives, and practitioner-patient relationships grounded in humility and listening, a different model of healing persists. One that prioritises presence over prescription. One that understands that trauma cannot be medicated away, that chronic illness cannot be solved without attending to environmental toxicity, and that suffering is not always a dysfunction—it is sometimes a form of protest. These spaces do not always look like "medicine." They may involve ritual, storytelling, movement, food, song, or silence. But they meet needs that standardised medicine cannot touch.

The future of healing lies in bridging these worlds. Not in replacing science with spirituality, nor in subordinating tradition to data, but in creating systems that honour both. This will require a radical shift—not just in practice, but in worldview. It will require acknowledging that health is not just a biomedical outcome, but a social, emotional, spiritual, and ecological condition. It will mean asking hard questions about who benefits from the current models, whose bodies are deemed worthy of care, and what kind of world we are trying to build when we talk about "health."

Until then, we live in the tension. A world where healing is both urgently needed and structurally marginalised. A world where health is sold back to us by the same systems that compromise it. In this context, reclaiming healing becomes a political and ethical act. It means remembering that your worth is not defined by productivity. That your symptoms are not failures, but signals. That healing, real healing, does not fit neatly into billing codes or business models. And that the body, despite everything, still knows what it needs—if only we are willing to listen.

The Myth of "Self-Care"

It is difficult to walk into a pharmacy, scroll through social media, or browse a modern bookshop without being inundated with the promise of self-care. Face masks, mindfulness apps, bath oils, sleep trackers, vitamin stacks—the wellness economy is saturated with products and protocols promising renewal, radiance, and resilience. Yet beneath the aesthetic lies a striking contradiction: never have we invested so much in the idea of care, and yet never have so many felt so depleted. The problem is not that people don't care for themselves. It's that the concept of self-care has been abstracted, sanitised, and ultimately commodified into something that has more to do with branding than with actual wellbeing.

The origins of "self-care" were radically different from its current form. The term gained prominence during the civil rights and feminist movements of the 1960s and 1970s, particularly among Black and marginalised communities. Self-care then was a political act—a way of preserving dignity and health under systems that devalued or endangered certain bodies. It was about survival in the face of systemic neglect. Audre Lorde, in her writing, famously insisted that self-care was not self-indulgence but "self-preservation, and that is an act of political warfare." The original framing was relational and resistant—rooted in community, justice, and reclamation. Today, that history has been largely erased from public memory, replaced by consumer-friendly versions of self-care that are more palatable to market logic.

This shift is not accidental. It reflects a broader cultural pattern in which collective strategies for survival are repackaged as individual lifestyle choices. The result is a narrative that subtly places the burden of healing entirely on the individual, while conveniently ignoring the structures that necessitate the need for such healing in the first place. If you are burnt out, anxious, or dysregulated, the problem—according to the self-care industry—is not that you live in a world of rising inequality, environmental degradation, racial violence, and overwork. The problem is that you haven't found the right adaptogen blend or taken enough digital detox weekends.

This reduction of care to consumer choice is not just superficial—it is structurally misleading. It reinforces the neoliberal assumption that health is an individual project, disconnected from social, economic, or ecological context. It implies that you can buy, schedule, or optimise your way into wellbeing if only you try hard enough. The logical extension of this belief is that if you are still unwell, still overwhelmed, or still exhausted, it must be your fault. You are not doing self-care correctly. You have failed to manage your time, your mind, or your body properly. This framing doesn't just miss the point—it compounds the very stress and shame it purports to alleviate.

Real care does not begin with consumption. It begins with rhythm, ritual, and relationship. It requires attention to what the body needs, not as prescribed by a wellness influencer, but as lived and felt through daily experience. That might mean slowing down when your culture insists on speeding up. It might mean prioritising sleep over productivity, food over fasting, or connection over performance. These are not glamorous acts. They do not yield immediate results. They cannot be posted as aesthetic achievements. But they restore integrity to the body and coherence to the nervous system.

One of the most overlooked aspects of true care is *interdependence*. The popularisation of self-care often omits this entirely. It romanticises solitude, personal space, and self-sufficiency, which are luxuries not equally accessible to all. Not everyone has the means to take a weekend away, hire a coach, or block out hours of uninterrupted silence. And even for those who do, the underlying belief that healing must be self-generated can be deeply alienating. The human nervous system does not regulate in isolation. It co-regulates. We are wired to calm, recover, and heal in connection with others—through shared meals, eye contact, physical touch, and safe presence. Any model of care that fails to account for this is not incomplete—it is inaccurate.

Ritual, too, is essential. Unlike routine, which is often imposed and mechanical, ritual is intentional and meaningful. It transforms the mundane into the sacred, the repetitive into the restorative. A morning cup of tea, if taken slowly and with reverence, can become a grounding act. The lighting of a candle at dusk can signal transition and integration. Simple acts, when done rhythmically and with presence, offer more to the nervous system than most curated wellness plans. Ritual reminds the body that it is held within time and meaning—not simply reacting to urgency, but attuned to continuity.

Rhythm is perhaps the deepest organising principle of true care. Our bodies function on rhythms—circadian, hormonal, seasonal. When we live against these rhythms, stress accumulates. When we honour them, repair becomes possible. Yet modern life is almost entirely structured to override rhythm. Workweeks ignore lunar cycles. Diets disregard natural hunger cues. Exercise is performed as punishment rather than pleasure. The goal of authentic self-care, then, is not to escape life but to resync with it. Not to achieve a curated image of balance, but to reinhabit the body's own temporal intelligence.

The implications of redefining care in this way are profound. It means shifting from performance to presence. From aesthetics to embodiment. From individualism to interdependence. It also means asking harder questions. What systems have taught us to associate rest with laziness? Why is slowness so often pathologised? What stories have we inherited about who is allowed to take up time, space, and softness? These are not ancillary questions. They are central to the ethics of care. Because without examining the narratives that shape our relationship to care, we risk replicating the very dynamics we're trying to heal from—power, perfectionism, productivity.

To move beyond the myth of self-care is not to abandon personal responsibility. It is to deepen it. It is to understand that caring for oneself cannot be separated from the conditions that make care possible. That health is not a solo pursuit, but a communal practice. That no face mask, however luxurious, can substitute for safety, belonging, or sleep. And that the most radical thing one might do, in a culture that sells healing as a product, is to reclaim care as something relational, rhythmic, and rooted.

There is nothing wrong with enjoying a massage, sipping herbal tea, or unplugging from screens. But if these acts are framed as the totality of care, they risk becoming distractions rather than tools. True care asks more of us—not in effort, but in honesty. It asks us to slow down not to escape the world, but to re-enter it with clearer boundaries and deeper presence. It reminds us that tending to ourselves is not about escaping responsibility, but about remembering what it feels like to be human—body, breath, heartbeat, relationship.

If we are to reclaim care from commodification, we must stop asking what to buy and start asking what to trust. What is sustainable? What is embodied? What returns us to rhythm, not rupture? The answers will not be sold to us. They must be remembered, rebuilt, and reinhabited—together.

Rest as Resistance

In a world that treats exhaustion as virtue and productivity as moral currency, rest becomes a radical act. This is not rhetorical flourish—it is political reality. To lie down without apology in a culture that worships overextension is to interrupt a centuries-long narrative of human value being equated with output. Rest challenges the foundational myths of modern capitalism: that time is money, that our worth is defined by our usefulness, that leisure must be earned, and that stillness is wasteful. These ideas are not neutral. They are ideological tools—historically developed, culturally embedded, and disproportionately harmful to those whose labour has been exploited, erased, or extracted under the guise of progress.

Tricia Hersey, founder of The Nap Ministry, brought this provocation to mainstream consciousness with clarity and force: *rest is resistance.* For Hersey, a Black woman theologian and performance artist, rest is not self-help; it is liberation work. Her assertion is that rest interrupts the machinery of white supremacy, patriarchy, and capitalism—systems that have systematically denied rest to those deemed less human, less worthy, less necessary. Hersey's invocation of rest is rooted in ancestral remembrance, not commercial wellness. It is spiritual, somatic, and historical—a reclamation of time, body, and dignity.

This reframing is particularly necessary because rest, as it is commonly understood, has been diluted into comfort-oriented consumerism. Plush robes, scented candles, and weekend retreats are marketed as rest but often serve as temporary compensations for unsustainable lives. The deeper work—the restoration of nervous system equilibrium, the reclaiming of internal rhythm, the undoing of inherited hypervigilance—rarely occurs in these contexts. What Hersey and other rest scholars highlight is that *rest is not the opposite of work—it is the interruption of domination.* It is the refusal to allow one's body to be used up for systems that do not serve one's thriving.

There is historical weight to this idea. Enslaved Africans in the Americas were denied rest as part of the systematised control of their bodies. Sleep deprivation was not incidental—it was enforced, woven into plantation economics and justified through pseudoscience and theology. The enforced sleeplessness of enslaved people is part of a broader lineage of labour control, one that continues in modern economies through shift work, wage precarity, and the glorification of "hustle culture." When Hersey says, "We will rest. We will not grind ourselves into dust," she is speaking to this intergenerational violence. Her work is not just poetic—it is forensic.

This framing challenges the universality often assumed in mainstream wellness discourse. Who can afford to rest? Who is punished for pausing? For whom is rest suspicious? These are not abstract questions. They play out in hospitals, classrooms, offices, and domestic spaces every day. A white tech worker who takes a sabbatical may be seen as enlightened; a Black woman who steps back from labour may be labelled lazy. A man who naps may be romanticised; a single mother who sleeps in may be judged. The right to rest is not equally distributed, and this inequality must be acknowledged if rest is to be reclaimed meaningfully.

Indigenous traditions across cultures have long held rest not as a reprieve from life, but as life itself. In many communities, rest is part of the cosmology. It is embedded in rituals, land-based practices, and seasonal rhythms. Among the Diné (Navajo), rest is relational—aligned with natural cycles and community wellbeing. In West African spiritual systems, rest is integral to spiritual hygiene, a means of keeping one's energy in alignment with the unseen world. Even in ancient Vedic traditions, rest was not idleness but an essential aspect of balance (*sattva*). These traditions treat rest not as an escape but as a gateway to clarity, creativity, and ethical living.

Contrast this with the modern Western view of rest as an accessory to productivity. Here, rest is useful only if it enables better output. Sleep becomes a biohack. Vacations are measured by their ROI in performance. Meditation is marketed as a way to sharpen focus, not soften presence. This instrumental view of rest fails to recognise that not all rest must serve a purpose beyond itself. Some rest is simply a return. A restoration of sovereignty over one's time and energy. A recalibration of the body's natural wisdom. This kind of rest resists metrics.

The physiological need for rest is often eclipsed by cultural pressure. Chronic stress leads to dysregulation of the hypothalamic-pituitary-adrenal (HPA) axis, altering cortisol rhythms and undermining immune and digestive function. Yet when people in states of collapse seek help, they are often given stimulants, told to exercise more, or encouraged to "power through." This advice stems from a system that refuses to recognise exhaustion as a valid endpoint. Burnout is medicalised, pathologised, or spiritualised—but rarely seen as a rational, adaptive signal that the current mode of living is unsustainable.

Rest, in this light, becomes diagnostic. Not in the clinical sense, but in the cultural sense. The inability to rest—whether due to internal guilt or external constraint—is data. It reveals how deeply one's nervous system has internalised the demands of extraction. Many people, even when given time off, cannot settle. Their body remains alert, breath shallow, mind restless. This is not laziness. It is survival. The body does not unlearn hypervigilance overnight. Rest must be *relearned.* And that relearning requires environments, practices, and relationships that are not governed by urgency.

What does it mean to create such environments? It means disrupting the social scripts that equate stillness with stagnation. It means recognising naps, pauses, and deep listening as legitimate forms of productivity—not in economic terms, but in human terms. It means restructuring institutions—schools, workplaces, faith spaces—to honour rest as a communal need, not a personal indulgence. The four-day workweek movement, universal basic income experiments, and trauma-informed education are all, in part, about re-centring rest. They reflect an understanding that sustainable contribution cannot happen in a state of constant depletion.

There is also an internal restructuring required. Many people carry shame about rest that has been passed down through generations. Their ancestors may have been denied rest; their parents may have equated rest with risk. To choose rest now may feel disloyal to those who had no such choice. This is where ritual becomes essential. Not the performance of rest, but the *practice* of it. Creating consistent, meaningful patterns of stillness—lighting a candle before sleep, walking without purpose, observing moments of silence after meals—can begin to rewire both the nervous system and the psyche.

To rest, then, is not simply to take a break. It is to reclaim a mode of being that resists commodification, domination, and depletion. It is to remember that we are not machines. That our worth is not tied to how much we produce. That rest is not the absence of action, but the presence of receptivity. And that healing—true healing—requires not more effort, but more space.

In reclaiming rest as resistance, we do not abandon responsibility. We realign with a deeper one: the responsibility to live in ways that honour our bodies, our histories, and our communities. We rest not to escape the world, but to return to it more whole. We rest to remember who we are beneath the noise. And we rest because, at the most fundamental level, rest is not a reward. *It is a right.*

Chapter 3
The Body Remembers the Way: Somatic Intelligence and the Wisdom Within

There is a quiet shift underway in our understanding of stress, trauma, and the nature of healing—not in laboratories or lecture halls, but in the very tissues that carry us. While our culture continues to place the crown on the intellect—championing positive thinking, mental resilience, and cognitive reframing—another truth, less showy yet far more elemental, has been steadily gathering weight. The body is not merely the site where stress announces itself. It is the language, the stage, and the speaker all at once. We do not hover above our bodies as impartial observers. We *are* our bodies. Until we grasp this—not as a pleasant theory but as a lived truth—mental insight alone will always fall short of dissolving the deeper imprints of strain. And so this exploration begins not with the mind's plans, but with the body's quiet genius: its ability to remember, to respond, and to repair—if we can bear to listen.

To say the body remembers is not poetic licence; it is biological, emotional, and sensory reality. Muscles clench in anticipation of threats that have long since passed. The breath tightens when we step into places that smell faintly of old anxiety. The stomach knots at the thought of exposure or rejection, as if bracing for a blow. These are not symbolic gestures. They are ancient, functional reflexes, born of an evolutionary pact to keep us alive. But when the danger recedes and the body remains on high alert—when the nervous system never quite gets the memo that "it's over"—we are left with chronic dysregulation. Not a personal failing, but the residue of unfinished survival responses.

This is where the idea of *somatic intelligence* steps in. It is the ability to notice and respond to the body's inner signals with a mix of accuracy and kindness—not through analysis, but through direct experience. Philosopher Eugene Gendlin, in his work on Focusing, gave us the term *felt sense* for this pre-verbal, intuitive knowing. It is not quite an emotion, not quite a thought. It might arrive as a tightening in the throat, a swell in the gut, a slight leaning forward in the chest—subtle signals whose meaning often resists language. In stress recovery, this kind of attunement is not decorative. It is central. Without it, healing remains a concept. With it, stress becomes less a battle to win and more a code to be deciphered.

The trouble is, our systems rarely teach this listening. Schools praise abstract reasoning. Offices reward quick wit and sharp intellect. Even therapy often stays tethered to words. The body, in the meantime, is treated as a kind of obedient vehicle—measured, medicated, even sculpted, but seldom consulted. Many can recite their diagnoses chapter and verse, yet have no words for the heaviness in their pelvis when they must choose, or the emptiness in their chest when they suppress grief. They know the names of their coping mechanisms but not the choreography of their survival patterns.

Relearning this language means relearning presence. Somatic tracking—a practice found in modern somatic therapies and in age-old contemplative traditions—is one way back. By observing sensation without rushing to change it, patterns start to appear. The lift of the shoulders before speaking. The subtle clench of the gut in the face of confrontation. The breath vanishing in a pause of uncertainty. These are not quirks; they are maps. Following them does not always lead to pain. Sometimes, it leads to the edge of release.

That the body stores emotional truth is hardly a new notion. In Traditional Chinese Medicine, the liver is linked to anger, the lungs to grief, the heart to joy, the kidneys to fear—patterns observed and refined over centuries. In Ayurveda, the doshas show similar affinities: Vata disturbances might echo as anxiety, Pitta as irritability, Kapha as a dampening of vitality. These frameworks agree on one thing: balance cannot be restored without addressing the emotions imprinted in the body's organs themselves.

Modern biomedical research, though more cautious in its language, is beginning to echo these insights. Studies of the enteric nervous system—sometimes called the body's "second brain"—and of the vagus nerve have reshaped our grasp of how physical and emotional regulation intertwine. Polyvagal theory tells us our nervous systems operate with a complex hierarchy, not a simple fight-or-flight switch. If the gut can register shame and the heart can register isolation, then healing must be more than talk. Breath, movement, touch, and sensory awareness are not optional extras; they are central routes back to balance.

Among these, breath deserves particular attention—not as a performance hack, but as a bridge between the voluntary and the involuntary. Most of us breathe in patterns we barely notice, each one carrying its own history. Breath that sits high in the chest can hint at vigilance. Fragmented inhalations and exhalations can whisper of trauma. A reluctance to fully exhale might speak of grief still held. Changing these rhythms is not as simple as "just breathe deeply." It can be an act of re-educating the nervous system, making space for safety to return. Breathwork, when handled with both care and precision, can free long-stuck survival energy, reawaken dulled areas of awareness, and knit back a sense of wholeness.

In some traditions, breath is more than physiology—it is spirit, *prana*, the pulse of life. Taoist and yogic teachings see its rhythms mirrored in the turning of seasons, the ebb of tides, the very cycle of birth and death. When we stop trying to dominate the breath and instead treat it as a teacher, the aim shifts. We are no longer just calming the mind; we are re-entering the body's natural rhythm.

But breath alone cannot untangle every knot. Movement matters. Many carry the debris of stress in the architecture of their muscles—jawlines locked by unsaid truths, hips braced by old violations, shoulders frozen in fear. These are not metaphors. They are physiological facts. And they often need a physical pathway out.

Dr David Berceli's Tension and Trauma Release Exercises (TRE) use neurogenic tremors—natural shaking generated deep within the body—to unlock this stored charge. The mind is not asked to narrate the trauma. The body is simply allowed to finish what it started long ago. Hands-on traditions, such as marma therapy in Ayurveda or craniosacral work in osteopathy, operate from the same premise: the practitioner listens with their hands, nudging the body towards release through resonance, not force.

Ultimately, the point is not to turn the body into another project to fix. It is to treat it as an ally, a witness, and—at times—the wiser of the two partners in our being. Stress, then, becomes less an enemy and more a courier. And the body, rather than a problem to be solved, becomes a library of memory and medicine.

The body remembers the path home. This is not metaphor; it is biology wrapped in lived experience. The question is whether we will finally be still enough to hear it. There are no shortcuts here, only the invitation to listen—to breath, to tremor, to the quiet intelligence in our tissues—and to begin again from that place.

Listening to the Felt Sense

It is entirely possible to go through life articulating your thoughts fluently, explaining your circumstances with rational clarity, and describing your emotional states with psychological accuracy—yet remain fundamentally disconnected from yourself. This disconnection is not a cognitive failure. It is a somatic absence: a lack of awareness of what the body is trying to say beneath the level of words. The concept of the "felt sense," introduced by philosopher and psychotherapist Eugene Gendlin, confronts this gap directly. The felt sense is not an emotion, not a sensation, not a thought—but a fusion of all three, forming a subtle, complex inner knowing that can only be accessed through patient attention. To listen to the felt sense is to enter into a deeper relationship with the truth of your lived experience. It is not mystical. It is neurologically grounded, psychologically profound, and therapeutically transformative.

Stress is often approached as a problem to solve or a dysfunction to manage. But when viewed through the lens of somatic tracking, stress reveals itself as information—encoded in the body, often incomplete, and always asking to be heard. A racing heart, a clenched jaw, a shallow breath, a sudden chill—these are not random artefacts. They are cues. They point to an inner environment shaped not just by the present, but by memory, conditioning, trauma, and expectation. The body, in this framework, is not a passive victim of stress. It is its historian. The felt sense allows us to access this history directly—not through intellectual analysis, but through embodied inquiry.

Somatic tracking is the practice of locating, observing, and gently engaging with the sensations and impressions that arise in the body in real time. It requires slowing down enough to notice what is usually bypassed: the tension behind a smile, the knot that appears before an email is opened, the flutter that follows a difficult conversation. The aim is not to fix or change these sensations, but to *attend* to them—to meet them with curiosity and care. This approach draws from multiple streams of knowledge: trauma-informed therapies such as Somatic Experiencing, mindfulness practices from contemplative traditions, and psychodynamic models of affect regulation. Despite their differing origins, they all converge on a single premise: *what the body holds, it can also resolve—if it is given attention, safety, and time.*

Many individuals operate with a fractured awareness of their own internal states. They may know, abstractly, that they are "stressed" or "burnt out," but cannot describe where or how that stress is felt. Ask them to locate the experience in the body, and there is a pause, a fumble, a vague answer: "in my shoulders, maybe?" This imprecision is not trivial. It reflects a disconnection from interoception—the ability to perceive internal bodily states, a foundational component of self-awareness. Neuroscience has shown that interoceptive pathways, primarily mediated through the insular cortex, play a crucial role in emotional regulation and self-coherence. When we track the felt sense, we are not engaging in a poetic exercise. We are stimulating and refining the neural circuits responsible for resilience, decision-making, and embodied presence.

Listening to the felt sense is not comfortable work. The body holds not only the wisdom of safety and longing but the residues of overwhelm, shame, grief, and fear. Often, the first sensations that arise are unpleasant. A tightness in the gut. A collapse in the chest.

A sense of heat, pressure, or emptiness. In conventional therapeutic models, these sensations may be interpreted as symptoms to regulate or reframe. In somatic work, they are portals. The discomfort is not a sign of failure. It is an invitation to go deeper. To feel the discomfort is not to indulge it but to metabolise it—to allow the body to process what the mind has avoided or the environment has suppressed.

This reorientation toward inner listening has implications beyond the individual. In high-stress professions—medicine, law, education, caregiving—the cost of chronic disembodiment is not just personal burnout but systemic breakdown. Workers become reactive, numb, or hypervigilant, operating from survival modes that narrow perception and inhibit empathy. When interoceptive capacity diminishes, so does the ability to attune to others. Compassion fatigue, often discussed in terms of over-giving, is more accurately understood as the consequence of disconnection from one's own needs. Somatic tracking, when embedded into daily rhythms, offers a corrective. A physician who takes thirty seconds between patients to scan their own body may notice fatigue in the eyes, tension in the jaw, or a subtle resistance to returning to the next task. That moment of noticing can become a moment of recalibration—shifting the entire tone of what follows.

Real-world applications of somatic awareness are already emerging in trauma-informed education, restorative justice practices, and leadership development. For example, in certain school settings, students are invited to track bodily sensations before responding to conflict—a practice that reduces impulsivity and deepens self-regulation. In conflict mediation, practitioners trained in somatic awareness can detect when a participant's body signals overwhelm—even before the person articulates it—and adjust the pace of dialogue accordingly. In boardrooms, executive coaches are teaching leaders to distinguish between urgency that arises from true insight and urgency that arises from stress reactivity. These are not soft skills. They are strategic competencies rooted in embodied intelligence.

There is also a deeper, more philosophical layer to the felt sense. In modern societies that valorise productivity and cognition, the body is often treated as a vehicle—instrumental, replaceable, and ultimately secondary to the mind. Listening to the felt sense reclaims the body as a source of meaning, not merely utility. It counters centuries of dualism that have separated mind from flesh, reason from instinct. When a person pauses to feel their body's response to a decision—whether to speak, to stay, to leave, to rest—they are engaging in a form of embodied ethics. They are consulting a compass that is older than language.

This doesn't mean the body is always right in some naïve, romantic sense. Trauma can distort perception. Chronic stress can create false alarms. But even distorted signals deserve to be heard. The purpose of somatic tracking is not to obey every sensation, but to *build a relationship* with it. Over time, this relationship matures. The person learns to discern between signals of genuine threat and echoes of past wounds. They begin to sense what "yes" and "no" feel like—not as concepts, but as physiological truths. They become less reactive, more responsive. Less fragmented, more integrated.

There is a quiet, subversive power in this work. It does not demand attention through performance or argument. It invites depth through presence. In a world that privileges explanation, somatic awareness values sensation. In cultures that reward speed, it rewards slowness. In systems that externalise healing, it restores the locus of wisdom to the individual—not as a siloed self, but as an embodied being in a relational world. When someone learns to listen to their felt sense, they are not only healing their own nervous system. They are subtly undermining the culture of dissociation that normalises burnout, hypervigilance, and disembodiment.

To begin this practice does not require special equipment, a retreat centre, or a wellness subscription. It requires a willingness to pause.

To sense. To befriend discomfort without rushing to solve it. To follow sensation as one might follow a thread in the dark—curious, patient, aware that it leads somewhere important even if the destination is not yet known.

In the long arc of healing from chronic stress, the felt sense is not a technique among many. It is the groundwork. It is where we return, again and again, to make sense of experience—not through ideas, but through presence. Not through explanation, but through attention. It teaches us that the roots of stress are not always found in the stories we tell ourselves, but in the sensations we have not yet learned to interpret. And that by listening—gently, persistently—we begin not just to heal, but to remember what it means to be fully alive.

The Organs That Speak Emotions

If you want to understand how stress lives in the body, don't start with the brain. Start with the liver. Or the gut. Or the lungs. In Traditional Chinese Medicine (TCM) and Ayurveda, stress is not just a psychological phenomenon—it is physiological, energetic, and organ-specific. These systems, developed over millennia through empirical observation and clinical refinement, articulate what modern medicine is only beginning to corroborate: *that organs are not silent cogs in a biological machine, but expressive centres of emotional and systemic intelligence.* Each organ carries patterns of response, memory, and meaning that shape how a person feels, reacts, and heals. And when stress becomes chronic, it doesn't simply float in the bloodstream as cortisol or adrenaline—it settles, embeds, and distorts function through specific pathways that these ancient systems have long charted.

Modern biomedicine has largely compartmentalised emotional states and physical organs, treating mental health and physical health as separate domains. Yet the data—neurological, immunological, and endocrinological—tell a more integrated story. For instance, the gut-brain axis reveals that disturbances in digestion influence mood and cognition via bidirectional signalling through the vagus nerve. Similarly, heart rate variability is now recognised as a key marker of resilience, emotion regulation, and trauma recovery. But while contemporary science builds its understanding from the outside in—studying mechanisms, molecules, and metrics—Ayurveda and TCM offer insight from the inside out, through the patient's lived experience.

In TCM, the liver is not just a metabolic organ. It is the seat of the free flow of qi (vital energy), associated with decisiveness, vision, and adaptability. When the liver becomes energetically stagnated—often due to repressed anger, unexpressed frustration, or the chronic suppression of personal boundaries—individuals may present with symptoms ranging from headaches and PMS to digestive disturbances and mood volatility. The language of "stagnation" may sound metaphorical to a Western ear, but the physiological correspondence is tangible: sympathetic overdrive, muscular tension, poor detoxification, and shallow breathing. Liver qi stagnation, in this light, is not poetic—it is diagnostic.

Ayurveda, with its tridoshic framework (vata, pitta, kapha), assigns the liver to pitta dosha—associated with fire, transformation, and digestion (both literal and metaphorical). When emotional fire is unmanaged—driven by ambition, anger, or inner heat—the liver becomes a crucible of burnout. This doesn't just manifest as irritability or overheating. It can lead to inflammatory conditions, skin flare-ups, sharp speech, and intensity that burns through relational harmony and internal peace. Practitioners learn to recognise the patterns: the executive with acid reflux and chronic impatience; the activist whose righteous anger curdles into cynicism; the student whose academic drive leaves them unable to rest. These are not pathologies of character. They are imbalances in organ systems shaped by emotional habit and societal conditioning.

The lungs, in both traditions, are organs of grief. In TCM, the lungs are responsible for taking in pure qi and releasing what no longer serves—both physiologically and emotionally. When someone experiences profound loss or unprocessed sorrow, it is not uncommon for respiratory function to falter. Breath becomes shallow, constrained, interrupted. Immunity weakens. The skin, also governed by the lungs in TCM, may become dull or hypersensitive. In Ayurvedic thought, the lungs are associated with kapha—the element of cohesion, structure, and emotional holding. When kapha becomes excessive, individuals may experience heaviness, withdrawal, mucus build-up, and emotional inertia. What looks like "laziness" or "fatigue" on the surface may be the physical echo of stored sadness.

The heart, revered across traditions as more than a pump, occupies a central place in the emotional topography of stress. TCM views the heart as the residence of the *shen*—the spirit, or conscious presence. A disturbed *shen* may manifest as insomnia, anxiety, forgetfulness, or incoherence in thought and speech. This is not merely symbolic. The connection between cardiovascular health and psychological distress is well-documented. Chronic loneliness increases risk for heart disease; emotional trauma can precipitate arrhythmias. But beyond pathophysiology, there is the subjective terrain: heartbreak, heartache, heart palpitations in panic, the felt sense of constriction during betrayal. TCM practitioners palpate the pulse not just for rate and rhythm but for subtleties in texture, tone, and resonance—seeking clues to emotional disruptions encoded in the heart's frequency.

In Ayurveda, the heart is the home of *sadhaka pitta*, a subdosha that governs mental clarity, emotional resilience, and the processing of sensory experience. A disturbed *sadhaka pitta* leads to a misalignment between perception and response. One might overreact to minor events, misread cues, or fluctuate between confidence and collapse. Such imbalances are not always traced back to trauma or psychological frameworks—they are read through digestion, sleep, and pulse. The Ayurvedic practitioner doesn't isolate the heart as an emotional centre alone, but observes its dialogue with the gut, the liver, the mind, and even the breath.

The gut, perhaps the most studied of these organs in Western research, serves as a bridge between ancient intuition and modern science. Ayurveda has long emphasised *agni*—the digestive fire—as central to health. If agni is weak, everything suffers: immunity, mood, clarity, even moral discernment. Unprocessed emotion is considered as dangerous as undigested food. In this paradigm, chronic stress impairs digestion not just by altering microbiota or peristalsis, but by disrupting the body's ability to discern and metabolise experience. TCM similarly associates the spleen (a key digestive organ in its system) with rumination, worry, and overthinking. When the digestive centre is overloaded—not just with food, but with thought—it collapses. Fatigue, bloating, brain fog, and emotional indecision are often linked to spleen qi deficiency, a condition that looks unremarkable on a lab report but is deeply felt by those who live with it.

One of the striking features of both Ayurvedic and TCM models is their relational logic. Organs do not operate in isolation, nor do emotions occur in a vacuum. The heart may be affected by the liver's heat, the lungs by the gut's sluggishness, the mind by the intestines' sensitivity. This systemic view is not merely elegant—it is clinically useful. A practitioner trained in these traditions listens differently. They listen to the story of the body as it speaks through organs, patterns, and pulses. They listen not just to what the patient says, but how the body says it—through tone, complexion, breath, posture, appetite, and response to touch.

Western medicine has made remarkable contributions in acute care, surgical precision, and molecular insight. But when it comes to chronic stress—the kind that eludes scans, bloodwork, and standardised assessments—its framework often falls short. A patient may be told they are "fine" despite living in a state of simmering distress. Labs normal. Vitals within range. Yet the individual feels off—uncentered, unmotivated, under attack from within. It is here that the wisdom of TCM and Ayurveda offers a crucial counterbalance: an invitation to *understand the body not as an object to be fixed, but as a subject to be listened to.*

This reorientation does not require abandoning science. It requires *expanding the definition of what counts as data.* In these traditions, sighing is data. Dream content is data. The colour of the tongue, the shape of the stool, the rhythm of the breath—all offer insights into how stress manifests, moves, and lingers. Healing, then, is not merely about suppressing symptoms or modifying behaviour. It is about restoring the body's expressive capacity—so that emotions can move through, rather than stagnate within.

To reclaim health through this lens is to enter into a relationship with one's organs as partners, not problems. The liver does not simply detoxify; it negotiates frustration and restraint. The lungs do not merely oxygenate; they grieve and release. The heart does not just beat; it loves, falters, and reorients. The gut does not just digest; it decides what is safe to hold and what must be let go. In the language of ancient medicine, these functions are not metaphorical—they are the ground upon which lasting healing stands.

Recognising this does not mean rejecting pharmacology or surgery when needed. It means no longer assuming that stress is generic, mental, or merely cognitive. It is precise. It is physiological. It has form, pattern, and location. And to address it effectively, one must speak the language of the body—not only in chemical terms, but in energetic, relational, and emotional ones. The organs are already speaking. The question is whether we are willing to listen.

The Breath as Healer, Not Just Tool

Breathing is the most democratic of human functions. It requires no permission, no tools, no technique. From the moment we emerge into the world until the last release of life, it accompanies us faithfully—often unnoticed, routinely undervalued. Yet, to reduce breath to a mere respiratory exchange is to overlook one of the most profound systems of healing, memory, and meaning available to the human experience. In nearly every ancient healing tradition, breath is not simply air moved in and out of the lungs—it is consciousness in motion. It shapes perception, stores history, and silently teaches us who we believe we are.

Modern wellness culture often positions breathwork as a technique, a stress hack, or an adjunct to yoga and mindfulness. But this instrumental view, while not inaccurate, is incomplete. When breath is reduced to a tool, it becomes something we do to manage our state—often in the service of performance, productivity, or temporary regulation. What this approach neglects is breath as a teacher of pattern, a mirror of identity, and a quiet historian of our inner life. *To breathe is not merely to stay alive—it is to express who we are at the level of the nervous system and beyond.*

The physiological impact of breath is well-documented. Respiratory rate influences heart rate variability, which in turn regulates autonomic balance between the sympathetic and parasympathetic branches of the nervous system. Fast, shallow breathing—a common default in high-stress states—activates the fight-or-flight response. Diaphragmatic, slow, and rhythmic breathing, conversely, signals safety and helps re-establish parasympathetic dominance. These observations, while useful, only scratch the surface. What is rarely asked is: *Why do certain individuals breathe shallowly even at rest? Why does the body resist deep inhalation in moments of perceived calm?*

The answers often lie not in mechanics, but in memory. Breath is a carrier of stored experience. People who have endured trauma, especially early developmental trauma, frequently develop breath-holding patterns as a way of surviving overwhelm. This is not a conscious decision—it is a form of physiological amnesia, a way of reducing sensory input to avoid emotional collapse. Over time, these patterns become invisible. The breath tightens not only in response to acute stress, but as a baseline orientation to the world. These individuals may not feel anxious, yet their respiratory patterns reflect an underlying vigilance. They have, quite literally, *forgotten how to breathe fully.*

In this sense, breath becomes identity. A person with a history of suppression may unconsciously limit the in-breath—struggling to receive, take up space, or expand emotionally. Another may have difficulty with the exhale—unable to let go, to release control, or to soften. These micro-habits are rarely taught in clinical settings, but somatic therapists, breathworkers, and trauma-informed practitioners observe them routinely. The breath doesn't lie. It broadcasts what the body knows, even when the mind has rationalised or forgotten.

Traditional systems of medicine understood this deeply. In yogic philosophy, the breath is prāṇa—life force—and every breath pattern is a reflection of one's inner alignment. The control of breath, or prāṇāyāma, is not merely a tool for lung health or mental calm, but a method of shaping consciousness itself. A scattered mind can be gathered through alternate nostril breathing; a restless body can be grounded through ujjayi. But even more fundamentally, breath was seen as the interface between form and formlessness—between the material and the subtle. It is no accident that nearly every meditation technique begins with attention to breath. It is the most accessible route back to now.

Chinese medicine, too, positions the breath at the heart of life force. The lungs are not only organs of respiration but the receivers of *heavenly qi.* Breath, in this view, is a spiritual as well as physiological act. Chronic sadness, grief, or unexpressed sorrow can literally lodge in the lungs, not just symbolically, but energetically—weakening defensive qi and compromising vitality. This is more than metaphor. It is a clinical observation: people who cannot grieve often suffer from bronchial issues, shallow breathing, or skin disorders (the lungs govern the skin in Traditional Chinese Medicine). The breath, therefore, becomes both messenger and medium.

What does it mean to move from technique to philosophy? It means approaching breath not just with manipulation, but with curiosity. Before instructing a client or patient to "take a deep breath," it may be more valuable to ask: *What is your breath doing right now? Where does it move? Where does it stop? What does it want to say?* This shift—from fixing to listening—can be quietly revolutionary. It acknowledges that the breath has its own intelligence, its own rhythm, and its own truth. Rather than imposing calm, we learn to discover what calm is obstructed by.

Consider the work of trauma therapist Peter Levine, whose somatic experiencing model frequently involves observing the breath's natural impulse to pause, expand, contract, or tremble during moments of deep integration. He notes that spontaneous changes in breath—sighs, gasps, or held inhales—often signal completion of a physiological stress cycle. These changes cannot be forced; they emerge when the body feels safe enough to let go. In this way, breath becomes a diagnostic tool—not something to control, but something to track with reverence.

Similarly, in the clinical application of breath in PTSD treatment, practices like coherent breathing (maintaining a consistent rhythm of around five breaths per minute) have been shown to restore autonomic regulation and reduce symptoms. But again, the most meaningful outcomes arise when these practices are taught not as drills but as invitations. The breath must be approached as a dialogue partner, not as a machine to be hacked.

There is also cultural wisdom in how breath has been treated across communities. In many Indigenous traditions, breath is integral to ritual. Songs, chants, and laments are breath-based technologies designed not only to express emotion but to move it through the body. Communal breathing—whether in singing, prayer, or movement—regulates nervous systems not just individually but collectively. The Western emphasis on solo breathing practices often misses this relational dimension. Breath, like healing, is rarely solitary.

Memory lives in the breath. Not only emotional memory, but generational. Epigenetic studies now suggest that trauma may leave biological traces in gene expression across generations. This may partly explain why certain breath patterns—especially breath-holding, irregular sighing, or difficulty with rhythm—are observed in families and lineages with histories of oppression, displacement, or chronic instability. Healing the breath, then, can become a form of ancestral repair. To breathe differently is not just to feel better—it is to embody a different story.

This also challenges the commercialisation of breathwork as a peak experience. Breath is not always cathartic. It doesn't always lead to bliss. Sometimes it leads to discomfort, sadness, resistance, or confusion. Sometimes the body coughs, trembles, or contracts when asked to breathe more deeply—not because it is broken, but because it is protecting. Breath, in this view, is not a linear path to calm. It is a spiral into sensation, a spiral into self. And like any meaningful practice, it requires patience, permission, and presence.

To treat breath as a healer, rather than a tool, is to restore its sovereignty. It means acknowledging that breathwork is not about imposing order, but about cultivating relationship. It means accepting that some breaths may be erratic, shallow, or guarded—and that these, too, are expressions of wisdom. It means reframing control as curiosity, and discipline as devotion.

Breath reveals the state of the nervous system more accurately than language. It also offers the most accessible intervention—non-invasive, non-pharmacological, always available. Yet its power lies not in how aggressively we can modulate it, but in how tenderly we can observe it. The breath, when treated with respect, becomes an oracle. It tells us what the body is ready for, what it is resisting, and what it remembers.

And so, the question becomes: *Are we willing to meet the breath on its own terms?* Can we be with it not to change it, but to understand it? Can we learn from its pauses, its tightness, its surges? To do so is to step into a different paradigm of healing—one that does not seek to override the body's intelligence but to trust it. This is the philosophy of breath not as escape, but as entrance—not as intervention, but as insight. And perhaps most powerfully, not as a performance of health, but as a return to wholeness.

Touch, Tremor, and Tension Release

If trauma lives in the body, then so too must healing. This foundational principle has begun to reshape not only somatic psychology and integrative medicine, but the very assumptions many people carry about recovery. For decades, emotional healing was largely confined to the terrain of the mind—words, insight, and cognition. But what if the most profound traumas are pre-verbal? What if the body remembers what the brain can't articulate? This is not metaphor. It is neurophysiological fact. *Touch, tremor, and tension release are not fringe tools—they are among the oldest, most primal forms of human regulation.*

In the increasingly crowded wellness landscape, one practice that has gained both empirical backing and anecdotal respect is Tension & Trauma Release Exercises (TRE). Developed by Dr. David Berceli, TRE is a somatic practice designed to activate the body's natural shaking mechanism to discharge stored stress and trauma. Rather than being seen as pathological, these tremors—often mild, rhythmic, and involuntary—are framed as *biological recovery responses*, similar to what animals in the wild exhibit after threat passes. They literally shake it off. Humans, however, have learned to override this process—due to social conditioning, shame, or chronic dissociation—leaving unresolved stress patterns frozen in musculature and connective tissue.

In practice, TRE involves a sequence of exercises that fatigue the major muscle groups, especially in the legs and pelvis, until neurogenic tremors are triggered—typically beginning in the psoas, a deep muscle linked to survival stress. These tremors are not dramatic or theatrical. They may present as a soft pulsing, a gentle vibration, or a subtle ripple along the spine. For many, the experience feels odd but relieving. Clients often report a sense of internal reset—like their nervous system has recalibrated without needing a story. This is crucial: *TRE bypasses narrative and restores regulation through physiology, not psychology.*

Consider the case of Daniel, a 45-year-old firefighter who had been living with low-grade anxiety and sleep disturbances for over a decade. Traditional talk therapy had helped to some degree, but it never fully alleviated the hypervigilance he felt in his body. During his third TRE session, Daniel experienced spontaneous tremors in his legs followed by what he described as "a strange wave of heat leaving my chest." He began to cry—not from sadness, but from what he called *recognition.* "It's like my body knew something I didn't," he later said. This type of embodied release—non-verbal, somatic, and emotionally integrative—illustrates what cognitive approaches often miss: *healing is not always linguistic.*

TRE is not a panacea, nor is it appropriate for everyone. People with complex trauma or dissociative disorders may require careful titration and professional supervision to avoid retraumatisation. But its power lies in its accessibility. It does not require analysis, performance, or conscious recall. It requires only presence, permission, and a body willing to move toward resolution on its own terms.

Parallel to the TRE paradigm is the ancient science of marma therapy, an Ayurvedic system of healing that works through touch—specifically, the stimulation of 107 energy points throughout the body where muscles, veins, ligaments, bones, and joints intersect. These marma points are not abstract constructs; they correlate closely with nerve junctions and lymphatic sites. When these points are gently pressed or massaged with herbal oils, they act as portals—releasing blocked energy, calming the nervous system, and restoring physiological balance.

In the West, marma therapy is often overshadowed by its cousin, acupuncture. But what distinguishes marma is its intentional softness. It doesn't penetrate; it listens. Marma practitioners speak of "unlocking the intelligence of the tissues," a phrase that points to the Ayurvedic belief that the body is not a machine but a *living archive of experience.* For instance, chronic anger may lodge in the liver marma; unresolved grief in the lung marma. Treatment is not just physical—it is relational. The practitioner meets the tissue with reverence, not force.

Take the example of Aarti, a 36-year-old woman recovering from post-viral fatigue and burnout. After six months of marma therapy, her energy levels had stabilised and her insomnia had abated. But what she emphasised most was the emotional effect: "It was like someone was finally listening to parts of me I didn't know were speaking." This echoes a truth often found in somatic work: *the body doesn't need to be fixed; it needs to be heard.*

Touch, in this context, is not superficial. It is diagnostic, therapeutic, and deeply sacred. Long before the advent of modern medicine, human beings touched each other to soothe, to diagnose, to transmit care. The mother who holds a fevered child, the midwife who presses on a labouring belly, the elder who blesses with a hand to the head—all of these acts contain knowledge deeper than instruction. Western clinical culture has largely medicalised or marginalised touch. Many physicians are now trained to minimise contact for fear of impropriety, litigation, or simple time constraints. But this has come at a cost: the nervous system craves safe, attuned touch as a core part of regulation. Its absence is not neutral—it is a form of deprivation.

Contemporary hands-on modalities, from craniosacral therapy to myofascial release, attempt to reclaim this lost dimension. Though differing in technique, they share a principle: *that healing often emerges not from intervention, but from attunement.* The practitioner listens through their hands, waiting for the tissue to guide them. In biodynamic craniosacral therapy, for example, the touch is featherlight—yet practitioners report shifts in breath patterns, autonomic tone, and even emotional release within minutes. Why? Because the body recognises safety when it is offered without agenda.

Even Western neuroscience has begun to affirm what traditional systems have long known. Oxytocin, often dubbed the "cuddle hormone," is released during safe touch and plays a key role in social bonding, stress reduction, and emotional repair. Studies also show that gentle touch activates C-tactile afferents—nerve fibres that specifically respond to affectionate, slow-pressure contact and send signals directly to brain regions involved in affective processing. These are not new insights. They are rediscoveries.

Touch, tremor, and tension release form a triad not because they are trendy, but because they access something primal. They offer pathways out of the cognitive dominance that often entraps trauma survivors in loops of explanation without integration. They speak to the language of the body—a language that predates speech, outlasts memory, and refuses pretense. They also remind us that presence—not performance—is the foundation of healing.

We live in a time when healing is often framed as something to be optimised, measured, and achieved. Yet the most enduring repairs often happen in silence, stillness, and subtle movement. A tremor that surfaces after decades of suppression. A marma point that finally lets go. A practitioner's palm resting without pressure, saying only: *I am here. You are safe.*

These are not dramatic interventions. But they are profound. Because they return us to something we didn't realise we had lost—

the capacity to be with ourselves without judgement, to meet the body not as an obstacle but as an oracle, and to understand that *true healing rarely arrives in the language of force.* It arrives in tremor. In touch. In the quiet release of what we were never meant to carry alone.

Chapter 4
Earth-Based Medicine: Naturopathy as Radical Remembrance

There is a certain irony—almost a quiet absurdity—in the way modern medicine now peers towards nature as though it were a curious novelty, a forgotten dispensary tucked away in the woods, or sunlight a newly unearthed "supplement." Yet nature has never been an optional extra. It is the original stage on which all life has played out. In contemporary usage, "natural healing" often means little more than swapping pills for herbs, creams for oils, or a daily walk for a prescription slip. But at its heart, naturopathy is not a game of replacements. It is a reorientation—a call to remember not merely what to take, but where we come from. This chapter approaches naturopathy as an act of radical remembering: not sentimental yearning for some romanticised past, but a conscious rewilding of body and mind within an ecological framework older than any clinic, older even than medicine as we know it.

Over time, the word "naturopathy" has been stretched thin—marketed into dilution by some, written off by biomedicine as fanciful or unscientific by others. Yet authentic naturopathy is not an adversary to conventional treatment; it is the context in which such treatment can sit more meaningfully. Mainstream healthcare tends to begin with the removal of symptoms. Naturopathy begins somewhere else—with the "terrain," both internal and external. It asks how lifestyle, environment, and estrangement from nature's rhythms set the stage for disease. The question shifts from "What will fix this?" to "What patterns, inside and around me, allowed this to take root?" Far from being an airy philosophical diversion, this is a clinical necessity in an age where disease is increasingly chronic, systemic, and fuelled by stress.

Industrial culture has conditioned us to see the body as a machine—something to be tuned, patched, or, in darker moods, simply managed. Naturopathy challenges this mechanical metaphor. It recognises the body as a living ecology, shaped and reshaped by light, food, weather, emotion, and place. Soil beneath the feet, the scent of plants, the touch of wind—these heal not only by chemical composition, but through relationship. Research increasingly validates what indigenous knowledge has long maintained: that the nervous system responds differently in the presence of trees; that contact with soil microbes enhances immunity; that living in step with daylight improves metabolic resilience. What was once dismissed as folklore is now couched in neurobiology—but the knowledge predates the words used to prove it.

One of naturopathy's quieter yet profound contributions lies in its attunement to rhythm—daily, seasonal, even generational. Where the modern world exalts unbroken productivity, naturopathic thought honours the ebb as much as the flow. Ayurveda's concept of ritucharya—seasonal living guided by environmental cues—is instructive here. Treatments are not fixed templates but are adapted to shifts in the doshas (vata, pitta, kapha) across the year. Traditional Chinese Medicine takes a parallel view, reading the body as a microcosm of five seasons, each paired with an organ and an emotional quality: spring with the liver and anger, autumn with the lungs and grief. In such traditions, healing is not about overriding change, but interpreting it—nature's own lexicon written into the body.

This rhythm is eroding in an age of artificial light, late-stage capitalism, and ecological detachment. Many live entire seasons indoors, experiencing sun through glass, eating food stripped of place and time. The loss is not just aesthetic—it is physiological. Disruption of the circadian clock is tied to a sweep of chronic conditions, from metabolic disease to depression. The remedy is not as simplistic as "more sunlight" or "eat seasonally." It is a wholesale redesign of how life is arranged, a return to principles that once underpinned health without conscious effort.

This is where the philosophy of naturopathy splits from its mass-market imitators. The modern wellness industry often sells "natural" in name only: essential oils in plastic bottles, adaptogens in capsules, organic fruit flown halfway around the globe. These may not be harmful, yet they obscure a truth: healing cannot be extracted, packaged, and sold in isolation. It must be cultivated, experienced, and engaged with in relationship. Treat plants merely as remedies, and they become commodities. See them as teachers, and they open a different kind of medicine—one grounded not in extraction, but in exchange.

Many contemporary herbalists and foragers are reclaiming this older approach—not merely using plants, but befriending them. Learning their cycles, their preferences, their habitats. Listening before harvesting. This is not sentimentality; it is clinical awareness. Plants produce compounds—alkaloids, terpenes, flavonoids—that vary with soil quality, weather patterns, and the stresses of their environment. Standardised extracts may offer measurable potency, but they sacrifice this ecological intelligence. A plant's medicine is never purely chemical; it is contextual.

Consider nettle (Urtica dioica)—prickly, assertive, mineral-rich. It offers iron and silica, supporting those with fatigue, anaemia, or connective tissue fragility. But herbalists know its medicine also lies in its character. It invigorates, awakens, sharpens boundaries for those blurred or dulled by chronic depletion. This tone comes from how nettle lives—vigorous, unyielding, thriving in disturbed ground. To take nettle is to take in its stance, not merely its nutrients.

This relational view echoes in the ancient practice of hydrotherapy. Cold immersions, river bathing, the rhythm of sauna and plunge, clay soaks—these are not Instagram-era novelties. They are ancestral technologies for recalibrating the body through deliberate engagement with elemental challenge and recovery. Science now explains how cold exposure activates brown fat, dampens inflammation, and steadies the autonomic nervous system. Yet standing knee-deep in a mountain stream is healing not only because of its temperature, but because it awakens a primal sensory world—sound, current, air, the feel of stone. It reopens a channel to what the body knew before fluorescent light.

Sunlight offers a similar lesson. Too often reduced to its role in vitamin D synthesis, it is, in truth, a master regulator—setting the circadian clock, influencing neurotransmitters, and shaping mitochondrial function. Heliotherapy, once a serious treatment for tuberculosis, skin disorders, and depression, disappeared not through lack of efficacy, but because it did not fit the machinery of modern healthcare economics. There is no profit in free light.

At the heart of naturopathy lies a reversal of the usual assumption: health is not something to be manufactured, but something already present, waiting for the right conditions to emerge. The role of the practitioner is not to impose health, but to create the ecological space in which it returns of its own accord. This is what makes naturopathy quietly radical—not in opposition to science, but in widening its frame, reminding us that we are not isolated mechanisms in need of repair, but embedded beings who have misplaced our sense of belonging.

This chapter will not hand over miracle cures or prescriptive regimens. Instead, it will trace the contours of another way of remembering—through season and soil, through plant allies and elemental therapies, through light and dark, work and rest. Each is a thread in a larger weave. Not to take us backward, but to bring us home.

Nature Is Not a Supplement: Rewilding the Body through the Roots of Naturopathy

It is no longer controversial to say that nature benefits health. Most people know that green spaces reduce anxiety, that sunshine improves mood, that walking in a forest lowers blood pressure. These truths have entered popular discourse, though often in the form of commodified advice: *Get more fresh air*, *Spend twenty minutes in nature*, *Take this adaptogen*. But what is rarely examined is the worldview beneath these prescriptions—the subtle assumption that nature is something we *use*, rather than something we *belong to*. Within much of modern wellness, nature has become a product: a supplement, a backdrop, a soothing balm to the discontents of civilisation. Naturopathy offers a deeper lens. It insists that healing does not come *from* nature in the way we receive pills from a pharmacy. It comes *through* our reintegration with it—as a process of rewilding, remembering, and realigning.

To understand naturopathy's radical potential, we must begin with its ecological roots. The term itself, from the Latin *natura* (birth, innate disposition) and Greek *pathos* (suffering, feeling), gestures toward an ethos where nature is not a lifestyle choice, but a foundational logic of health. Early naturopathic practitioners in 19th-century Europe—figures like Sebastian Kneipp, Benedict Lust, and Louis Kuhne—were not seeking to create a gentler version of medicine. They were reacting to the mechanistic worldview of industrial science, which had begun to treat the body as a sealed apparatus, isolated from its habitat. Their core insight was deceptively simple: that disease is not an isolated event, but a systemic dissonance—between person and place, lifestyle and land.

This insight places naturopathy firmly in the tradition of ecological medicine. It does not seek to dominate symptoms but to observe patterns. The body is not broken, it is *out of sync*—disoriented by environments that no longer nourish, rhythms that no longer flow. The naturopath asks not just what hurts, but what is missing. This is a fundamentally different diagnostic frame from biomedicine's pathology-centred model. Where the latter searches for biochemical errors, naturopathy looks for interrupted relationships: to food, to rest, to seasonality, to sunlight, to emotion, to ancestry. In this context, "natural" is not shorthand for "plant-based" or "chemical-free." It refers to *the context in which life evolved to flourish.*

Yet this vision has been repeatedly diluted—especially in the commercial wellness industry, which frequently reduces nature to a menu of products and protocols. The rebranding of ancient herbal traditions into marketable tinctures, the appropriation of indigenous wisdom into detox kits, the reduction of soil-based immunity into probiotic pills—these trends strip natural medicine of its *relational intelligence.* Authentic naturopathy does not ask how we can extract nature's benefits. It asks how we can *re-enter a participatory relationship with the living world.* It is not about taking the forest into the pharmacy, but about recognising the pharmacy within the forest.

This distinction becomes critical when we consider how the body itself evolved. Our physiology is not adapted to modern schedules or built environments. It evolved in synchrony with circadian light patterns, in microbial intimacy with soil, in sensory dialogue with the land. When we live in sealed buildings, surrounded by processed food, neon light, and digital input, our systems are not simply deprived—they are confused. Chronic inflammation, autoimmune conditions, hormonal imbalances, and nervous system dysregulation are not random flaws. They are *adaptive responses to maladaptive environments.*

Rewilding, then, is not a lifestyle trend. It is a clinical imperative. And in naturopathic terms, rewilding refers not to abandoning the modern world, but to reanimating the body's original intelligence. This might mean walking barefoot on earth not as a novelty, but as a method of electrical grounding—now supported by studies showing reductions in cortisol and systemic inflammation. It might mean cold water exposure not as a performance hack, but as a way of reawakening vascular tone and resilience. It might mean treating mealtimes not as fuel stops but as seasonal rituals—eating what grows near, what grows now, and what grows cleanly.

One of the most powerful expressions of this ethos can be seen in the rhythms of traditional food cultures. In Sardinia, Okinawa, and the Nicoya Peninsula—places noted for longevity—people do not "supplement" with nature. They live within it. Their diets are not constructed by nutritional data but by agricultural rhythms. Their movement is not structured through fitness apps but through manual life. Their rest is not optimised but taken in alignment with the sun and silence. The body is not managed, it is *entrained.* And this entrainment—the synchrony between body and biosphere—is what modern environments have so thoroughly disrupted.

Naturopathy restores this synchrony through practice, not prescription. It is not enough to advise a person to "spend more time in nature" without addressing the systemic barriers that make this difficult. The nature-deficit disorder is not merely personal—it is architectural, economic, political. Public parks are sparse in low-income areas. Working hours often prevent daylight exposure. Urban planning routinely severs communities from water, trees, and sky. Any serious vision of natural healing must therefore be structural, not just individual. Rewilding the body implies rewilding society.

Yet the temptation remains to isolate nature's "active ingredients" and market them back to the public. This is where we must be vigilant. When chlorophyll becomes a commodity, or forest air is sold in canisters, we are no longer engaging with nature—we are consuming its fragments. The illusion of wellness is maintained, but the ecology of healing is lost. True naturopathic practice refuses this fragmentation. It holds that healing occurs not from substances, but from *conditions*. Just as a plant needs not only water but the right soil, so the human system needs more than supplements—it needs *contextual coherence.*

This coherence is profoundly somatic. It is felt when the sun warms the skin, when the wind touches the face, when soil is smelled, when birdcall replaces the hum of traffic. These are not poetic embellishments; they are sensory inputs with measurable effects on the nervous system. Research in psychoneuroimmunology has shown that environments rich in biodiversity reduce markers of stress, enhance immune surveillance, and modulate inflammatory pathways. But the deeper implication is this: *nature is not therapeutic because it is relaxing. It is therapeutic because it is familiar.* Our bodies recognise it not as novelty, but as home.

This article is not a call to reject science. It is a call to *expand* it—beyond laboratories, beyond market algorithms, into the forests, kitchens, gardens, and rivers where healing has always taken place. Naturopathy does not oppose evidence. It insists on more inclusive evidence—evidence that honours complexity, relationships, stories, and the subtle feedback loops between body and biome. To reduce healing to data alone is to ignore half the equation. The body does not only respond to what it consumes. It responds to where it *belongs*.

Nature is not a supplement. It is the original condition. And to treat it as accessory—as a side note to medicine—is not just ecologically naive. It is biologically incoherent. As rates of burnout, autoimmune illness, metabolic dysfunction, and chronic fatigue rise, the question we must ask is not what pill to take, but *what pattern have we broken*? Naturopathy answers with clarity: the pattern of relationship—to land, to time, to rhythm, to breath, to food, to the living world.

The articles and practices that follow in this chapter are not new discoveries. They are ancient invitations—renewed. They speak to the part of the reader that is not just a patient, not just a consumer, but a body that remembers forests, a gut that recognises soil, a skin that still yearns for sun. Healing, in this light, is not the result of intervention. It is the result of *re-inhabiting a world we never truly left, only forgot how to feel.*

The Healing Pulse of the Seasons: Circadian and Seasonal Living Across Cultures

Modern health advice often reduces time to a scheduling issue—optimise your morning routine, block your calendar, manage sleep with a wearable device. Yet deep within many traditional healing systems lies a more fundamental proposition: that health is not merely something we *do* in time, but something that emerges when we *align* with it. Time, in this context, is not clockwork—it is cyclical, ecological, and embodied. The body is not a machine operating independently of its surroundings; it is a rhythmic organism pulsing in concert with day, night, moon, tide, soil, and season. To forget these rhythms is not just a poetic loss—it is a physiological disruption. Circadian and seasonal disconnection may be one of the most under-recognised contributors to chronic illness in industrial societies.

The circadian system, once relegated to sleep research, has now emerged as a central regulatory network of nearly every biological process. Governed by light-sensitive cells in the suprachiasmatic nucleus of the brain, our internal clocks coordinate everything from cortisol production to immune surveillance, gut motility to gene expression. Yet these clocks are not autonomous. They are entrained by environmental signals—sunlight, temperature, food timing, activity, and social cues. When these cues become chaotic, misaligned, or absent—as they often are in artificial lighting, shift work, jet lag, or digital immersion—the circadian architecture begins to fray. What results is not an isolated symptom, but a systemic disorientation: insomnia, hormonal imbalances, depression, inflammation, and metabolic syndrome.

This insight is not new. Long before the language of chronobiology emerged, traditional medicine systems designed entire therapeutic frameworks around time. In Ayurveda, *dinacharya* (daily rhythm) and *ritucharya* (seasonal rhythm) are foundational. Each hour of the day is assigned a doshic influence—vata, pitta, or kapha—and specific behaviours are recommended accordingly: early rising before sunrise, main meal at solar noon, gentle wind-down after sunset. Likewise, the seasons are seen not simply as changes in weather but as shifts in elemental forces. Autumn's dryness demands oiling and grounding foods; spring's dampness calls for cleansing and stimulation. These are not superstitions—they are refined empirical observations of how the human body responds to environmental flux.

Traditional Chinese Medicine (TCM) also exemplifies this seasonal intelligence. Each organ system corresponds to a season: the liver with spring, the heart with summer, the lungs with autumn, and the kidneys with winter. These associations are not metaphoric. They reflect a recognition that biological energy (qi) moves differently across time. For example, spring is seen as the time of liver qi expansion—an ideal period for movement, emotional release, and detoxification. Winter, associated with the kidneys, invites conservation, rest, and warming practices. To ignore these patterns, from a TCM perspective, is to work against nature's current—to strain vitality rather than cultivate it.

In both systems, food is not simply a source of calories but a carrier of seasonal intelligence. Eating root vegetables in winter, bitter greens in spring, hydrating fruits in summer, and warming stews in autumn is not a culinary trend but a way of informing the body about its place in time. The Western nutrition model, with its emphasis on macronutrients and caloric balance, often overlooks this temporal dimension. Yet when we eat strawberries in December, or tomatoes shipped across continents, we are not just consuming out-of-season produce—we are confusing the biochemical cues that align digestion, immunity, and hormone cycles with the Earth's rhythms.

Circadian disruption is not only a personal matter; it is a cultural architecture. The 24/7 economy, artificial lighting, blue screens, shift work, and decoupling from natural cycles create a kind of temporal exile. This is not a metaphor—it has measurable impacts. Studies have shown that shift workers have significantly higher risks of cardiovascular disease, diabetes, and cancer. Children exposed to excessive artificial light exhibit altered melatonin rhythms. Even small misalignments between sleep timing and biological clocks—what researchers call "social jet lag"—have been linked to weight gain, depression, and reduced cognitive function.

But the damage is not only physiological. It is relational. Our sense of belonging—both to ourselves and to our environment—is mediated by time. Rituals rooted in seasonality, such as solstice festivals, harvest gatherings, and planting ceremonies, historically served to synchronise not only internal rhythms but social coherence. As these rituals vanish or become commercialised, what is lost is not only tradition—it is entrainment. The body no longer knows when to rise, when to rest, when to eat, when to release. Healing, in this context, becomes a matter of re-synchronisation.

This re-synchronisation is not achieved by downloading another app. It is achieved through what philosopher Ivan Illich once called *tools for conviviality*—practices that restore rhythm without demanding performance. Waking with natural light, walking at dusk, eating meals outdoors, observing moon phases, taking seasonal sabbaths, lighting candles after sunset, fasting with equinoxes—these are not quaint customs, but methods of re-attunement. They activate what neurobiologist Stephen Porges describes as "neuroception of safety"—the body's ability to detect environmental coherence and shift into parasympathetic restoration.

These practices have modern applications. In integrative medicine, circadian-based interventions are gaining traction. Time-restricted eating, for instance, shows benefits for metabolic health not solely due to caloric restriction, but because it aligns feeding with the body's natural insulin sensitivity curve. Likewise, "chrono-therapy" in psychiatry leverages sleep phase adjustment to treat depression. Even cancer therapies now increasingly consider the timing of drug delivery to optimise efficacy and minimise side effects. What we are witnessing is not the invention of new wisdom, but the rediscovery of ancient patterns—translated into contemporary language.

Yet if we limit this conversation to biology alone, we risk stripping it of its deeper significance. Seasonal living is not just about preventing disease. It is about cultivating coherence—between inner and outer time. It affirms that the body is not a container, but a participant in Earth's unfolding rhythm. When a person aligns with light and dark, heat and cold, expansion and contraction, they are not just healthier—they are more *whole*. Illness, from this view, is not only a failure of cells or systems, but often a sign of separation—from pace, from place, from pattern.

This insight is particularly vital in an age defined by acceleration. In the high-speed tempo of digital life, where emails arrive without time zones and artificial light flattens day and night, the body loses its bearings. Fatigue, anxiety, and burnout are not individual weaknesses—they are circadian injuries. The call to seasonal and circadian living, then, is not nostalgic. It is revolutionary. It challenges the dominant economic logic that time is money, and reclaims time as *medicine.*

Different cultures have guarded this medicine in diverse ways. In Japan, the concept of *shinrin-yoku* (forest bathing) invites people to immerse themselves in woodland environments not for exercise, but for sensory restoration. In Nordic countries, *hygge* and *koselig* valorise winter slowness—candles, blankets, warm food—as survival wisdom. Among Andean communities, seasonal festivals like *Inti Raymi* honour solar cycles through communal ritual. In Jewish tradition, *Shabbat* is a weekly reset that affirms sacred rest. These practices are not luxuries. They are technologies of rhythm.

Modern medicine, for all its progress, has largely ignored rhythm as a therapeutic axis. It measures, it diagnoses, it treats. But it rarely asks when. When should the body rest? When should it move? When is the right time to grieve, to fast, to cleanse, to create? The healing pulse of the seasons provides a framework for these questions. It offers not just prescriptions, but *permissions*—to slow down in winter, to rise in spring, to exhale in autumn. It reminds us that wellness is not static; it is *seasonal intelligence embodied.*

To restore this intelligence is not merely a lifestyle tweak. It is an act of ecological reintegration. In aligning with the sun's arc and the soil's cycle, we remember what the nervous system has always known: that we are time-sensitive creatures, and that healing is not a protocol but a pattern—a returning to the pulse we were born to follow. The following sections will explore how these pulses manifest in breath, in food, in temperature, and in emotion. But the foundation is this: to heal in rhythm is to return to rhythm—not as a technique, but as a way of being that makes sense not just to the intellect, but to the cells themselves.

Plants as Relationship, Not Remedy

Modern herbalism is increasingly framed in clinical terms—tinctures measured in millilitres, capsules stacked on wellness shelves, and plant extracts fitted into symptom-treatment algorithms that mimic pharmaceutical logic. But this mechanised view obscures a deeper lineage. For most of human history, medicinal plants were not isolated ingredients; they were living beings in relationship with those who tended, harvested, and prepared them. To reduce plant medicine to a pill is not merely a simplification—it is a rupture from a worldview in which healing was as much about reciprocity as it was about remedy. *To know a plant was to know its season, its temperament, its terrain, and the stories it carried.*

In many traditional systems, plants are not passive substances to be extracted. They are animate teachers, shaped by soil, sky, and symbiosis. Among Indigenous communities—whether Andean, Maasai, or Anishinaabe—plants are approached with ceremony, not commodification. Before harvesting, there may be offerings. Before ingestion, there is often prayer. These are not quaint rituals; they are epistemological practices—ways of affirming that healing is relational, and that wellness cannot be extracted from context. *The very act of using a plant for medicine traditionally implied a responsibility to its ecosystem.*

This ethos is largely absent from the industrialised wellness industry. In many Western contexts, herbal supplements are marketed with the same language of biohacking and optimisation that governs nootropics and protein powders. "Take as needed" implies a one-way relationship. But plants are not drugs. Their efficacy cannot be fully understood without also accounting for rhythm, ritual, and respect. The same valerian root, for example, may calm one person and agitate another—not because of biochemical error, but because the body's receptivity depends on constitution, context, and seasonal timing. This variability is not a flaw; it is a reflection of the living nature of both plant and person.

Rachel Corby, a British plant spirit healer, describes her practice not in terms of extraction, but conversation. "I don't 'use' plants," she says. "I listen to them." Her work involves sitting with a plant for hours—sometimes days—without ingesting it, simply observing its form, fragrance, growth pattern, and energetic signature. This may sound esoteric to a pharmacologist, but it is not unlike what ethnobotanists do in fieldwork or what traditional Chinese herbalists are trained to discern. Observation, presence, and intuition are part of the diagnostic palette—*not because science is rejected, but because the plant is not reduced.*

Similarly, Irish herbalist Jo Dunbar notes that many clients seeking herbal remedies are surprised when the first consultation includes questions about dreams, grief, and ancestral stories. "A good herbal formula is not just about symptom matching," she explains. "It's about alignment. What is this person trying to metabolise emotionally? What is unresolved in their terrain—inner and outer?" Her use of hawthorn, for instance, is never generic. For a person with heart palpitations and deep loneliness, she may combine it with rose and motherwort, not because a textbook says so, but because the relational qualities of the plants support the client's energetic profile.

These nuances are lost in standardised extracts and globalised supply chains. When turmeric becomes a global supplement trend, its relational depth—its place in Indian kitchens, in religious rituals, in the collective memory of grandmothers—is flattened. As herbalist and author Rosalee de la Forêt warns, "We don't need to exoticise plants from halfway across the world. Often, the best medicines are growing right outside our door." Her approach encourages people to learn local flora, to forage ethically, and to remember that *place matters*. Healing is not imported; it is rooted.

There is also a growing movement among foragers and herbalists to resist the commodification of endangered plants. Goldenseal, American ginseng, and chaga are now under threat not because of traditional use, but because of unsustainable harvesting driven by demand from wellness consumers unaware of ecological impact. In this context, ethical herbalism becomes not just a matter of sourcing, but of worldview. Does the practice reinforce extraction, or does it regenerate relationship?

In the Andean highlands, the practice of *ayni*—sacred reciprocity—guides all plant interactions. One does not harvest without giving back. This might involve composting, planting companion species, or offering water to the roots. In Amazonian traditions, working with psychoactive plants like ayahuasca or tobacco involves strict dietary, energetic, and social protocols—not as superstition, but as acknowledgment that the plant is a conscious being. One enters into its domain humbly, not with entitlement.

There is a tension here worth examining. Scientific herbalism has brought legitimacy to plant medicine in clinical settings. Trials, standardisation, and pharmacological understanding are crucial in ensuring safety and efficacy. Yet when this approach dominates, it can eclipse the more relational and ritualistic frameworks that gave plant medicine its depth to begin with. *The challenge is not to choose between science and spirit, but to hold both—to value biochemical constituents and ecological relationships as equally important.*

Plants also have emotional and spiritual intelligences that defy reduction. Grief, for example, is not a diagnosis, yet it often underlies physiological complaints. In many traditions, mugwort is used not just for digestion but for dreamwork, for accessing repressed memory, for journeying between realms. Lavender is more than a sedative—it is a balm for frayed spiritual edges. When we approach plants with reverence, they often work beyond our expectations. They do not simply target symptoms; they *tune* the whole.

Modern mental health practitioners are beginning to recognise this. In somatic therapy, herbs are sometimes used not for their pharmacodynamics but for their symbolic resonance. A client working through boundary issues might be invited to sit with nettle—not ingesting it, but noticing its sting, its firmness, its clarity. This is not placebo; it is *relational metaphor made somatic.* The plant becomes a teacher, not a product.

The resurgence of community herbalism—seeded through apothecaries, mutual aid projects, and land-based healing collectives—is part of a wider reclaiming of health sovereignty. These spaces often prioritise ancestral knowledge, community access, and ecological justice over profit. They restore herbal medicine to its original domain—not the supplement aisle, but the commons. Plants in this context are not peddled as quick fixes. They are companions in a process of reconnection: to land, lineage, and self.

To treat plants merely as remedies is to replicate the logic of the pharmaceutical model—where health is a commodity, and healing is outsourced. But to engage with them as relationships requires time, listening, and reciprocity. It reframes healing as a co-created process: not *what can this plant do for me*, but *what kind of relationship can we form?* This is a subtler, slower path. But it is also more enduring.

The language we use matters. When we say "this herb *treats* anxiety," we place it in a mechanistic frame. But when we say "this plant supports the nervous system, soothes the heart, and invites calm," we are speaking in terms of *relationship*. It is the difference between command and collaboration. Between extraction and invitation. Between control and communion.

As herbalist Asia Suler writes, "The plants are not here to save us. They are here to *remember* with us." This remembering is not nostalgic—it is radical. It reorients healing from the clinic to the forest floor, from the expert to the ecosystem, from the pill bottle to the open hand. It reminds us that to heal with plants is to enter into dialogue—not with a substance, but with a living intelligence shaped by millennia of sun, soil, and survival.

And perhaps that is the most powerful medicine of all—not what a plant does to us, but what it *asks of us*: to slow down, to pay attention, to belong. When we accept that invitation, we do not merely "use" plants. We learn from them. We heal *with* them. And in doing so, we heal something much older than illness—we heal the rupture between body and Earth.

Water, Sun, and Soil: The Forgotten Medicines

If the word "medicine" instinctively conjures a pill or prescription, we are already speaking from within a worldview that is historically narrow and industrially engineered. The deeper lexicon of healing—one grounded in lived human biology, ancestral knowledge, and planetary rhythms—once included the elements themselves: *water, sunlight, and soil.* These were not seen as passive backdrops to life, but as *active agents of health,* capable of restoring, recalibrating, and remembering the body into balance. That modern medicine has largely relegated them to the periphery—as lifestyle advice, not therapeutic intervention—is both telling and costly. What has been dismissed as quaint is, in many traditions, the foundation of resilience.

Water, sun, and earth have always been part of the original pharmacopeia, long before chemistry claimed authority over wellness. The shift away from these elemental therapies is less a scientific evolution than a cultural amnesia—a forgetting fuelled by profit models that cannot patent sunlight or package a barefoot walk. *To restore these medicines to their rightful place is not anti-science; it is anti-forgetfulness.* It is a return to ecological memory in a time of profound physiological disconnect.

Hydrotherapy, for instance, is often misunderstood as either spa luxury or folk superstition. But its roots are clinical and rigorous. In 19th-century Europe, water therapy was the backbone of several medical systems, including the famed Kneipp method developed by Bavarian priest Sebastian Kneipp. His approach integrated alternating hot and cold water exposure, barefoot walking, and immersion in rivers—anchored by a belief in the body's innate capacity to self-regulate when stimulated correctly. These were not indulgences. They were prescriptions.

Modern research affirms what was once observational knowledge. Cold-water immersion has been shown to modulate the vagus nerve, lower systemic inflammation, and improve immune function. Thermoregulation through saunas, another legacy practice, correlates with cardiovascular benefits and reduced all-cause mortality. The Finnish sauna is not a wellness fad; it is a national health intervention. What matters is *consistency, context, and cultural framing.* Hydrotherapy is not a one-off trick. It is a patterned conversation with the nervous system—one that teaches the body how to recalibrate between extremes.

Yet in clinical settings, water's role has become marginal. Few hospitals prescribe therapeutic bathing. Few general practitioners understand hydrotherapy as a legitimate protocol. Instead, patients are told to hydrate and, at best, encouraged to take a walk. The elemental intelligence of water—its weight, its temperature, its kinetic pull—is ignored. And so are its emotional dimensions. Across cultures, water rituals have always been tied to grief, purification, and release. To enter water is to surrender. To emerge is to begin again.

Sunlight faces a similar paradox. On one hand, dermatological culture has pathologised sun exposure through decades of fear-based messaging around skin cancer. On the other, the surge in vitamin D deficiencies—linked to immune dysregulation, depression, and metabolic disorders—reveals a population chronically under-exposed to light. We have designed entire cities that make it easier to charge a phone than to receive natural light on the skin.

But sunlight is not simply about vitamin D. *It is a circadian signal.* The body's hormonal rhythms—cortisol awakening response, melatonin release, insulin sensitivity—are all entrained by exposure to morning light. Photoreceptors in the eyes and skin communicate directly with the suprachiasmatic nucleus, the brain's internal clock. Light is not cosmetic; it is *instructional.* Without it, the body loses temporal coherence. Jet lag, shift work, and excessive screen exposure are all forms of circadian injury.

This makes the timing and quality of light exposure a legitimate therapeutic intervention. Emerging fields like chronobiology and circadian medicine now advocate for sunlight as a first-line input in treating sleep disorders, depression, and even cancer. But again, this knowledge is not new. Ayurveda has long recognised the *dinacharya*—a daily routine aligned with solar rhythms. Indigenous healing traditions across continents have aligned rituals with dawn and dusk. *To synchronise with the sun is not a lifestyle choice; it is a form of biological diplomacy.*

Then there is the earth itself—our most intimate, neglected contact zone. Most modern humans spend the majority of their lives in shoes, on concrete, inside climate-controlled buildings. This detachment from soil is not just physical; it is neurological. Direct skin contact with the ground—often called "earthing" or "grounding"—has been shown in small but promising studies to reduce markers of inflammation, improve heart rate variability, and support wound healing. The proposed mechanism is electrical: the Earth carries a subtle negative charge, which may neutralise oxidative stress in the body. Critics dismiss this as fringe. But *no one denies that we are electrical beings.* The idea that the Earth's charge might affect us is not mystical—it is mechanistic.

More provocatively, soil is also microbial medicine. The "hygiene hypothesis" posits that exposure to diverse soil bacteria in early life trains the immune system to respond appropriately to threats. Children raised on farms, for example, exhibit lower rates of asthma and allergies—a correlation backed by decades of epidemiological data. Soil is not dirty; it is *developmental.* And our disconnection from it is manifesting in immune confusion.

These three forgotten medicines—water, sunlight, and soil—are not separate. They form a triad of environmental intelligence that continuously informs human physiology. In nature-based medical systems, their use is seasonal, personalised, and ritualised. A morning sunbath in winter, a river soak in spring, a barefoot walk through summer soil—each of these is a practice, a pulse, a prescription. The problem arises when we remove them from their context, reduce them to wellness content, or skip their relational component entirely.

Real-world examples illustrate this more vividly than theory. In northern Thailand, hill tribe communities use smoke and steam from boiled herbs in postpartum care—a ritual combining water, heat, and plants to cleanse and strengthen. In Japanese *shinrin-yoku* (forest bathing), sunlight filtered through leaves combines with terpenes from trees to lower cortisol and boost immunity. In Nordic countries, cold plunges in icy lakes followed by sauna rituals recalibrate stress responses. These are not luxury experiences. They are community-sanctioned medicine.

Contrast this with the Western wellness landscape, where infrared saunas and blue-light blocking glasses are sold without narrative, context, or cultural memory. The body may respond physiologically, but something vital is lost in translation. The ritual dimension—the part that says, "this act connects me to land, lineage, and life"—is amputated. Without it, we risk turning ancient medicine into modern distraction.

There is also a moral imperative here. Reclaiming elemental therapies is not just about personal healing. It is about ecological remembering. If we treat water, sun, and soil as medicines, then pollution, deforestation, and climate instability are not abstract crises—they are attacks on the foundations of health. To advocate for clean rivers is not just environmentalism; it is *clinical urgency*. To protect old-growth forests is to defend a pharmacopoeia that no lab could replicate.

This reframe also demands humility from practitioners. No supplement, however advanced, can replace an hour in the forest. No app can deliver the recalibration of an ocean swim. And no protocol can override the body's ancient attunement to Earth rhythms. To ignore this is to medicalise a symptom and miss the source. To remember it is to move from intervention to integration.

We must also reconsider the metrics of efficacy. Water, sun, and soil do not promise immediate relief. Their power lies in their *accumulated fidelity*. They are slow medicines, quiet tutors, and precise mirrors. They teach through consistency. A daily walk at dawn may not rival the drama of a new diagnosis, but over years, it changes the body's architecture—*not just its symptoms, but its sense of being.*

In a culture that measures healing in speed and visibility, these therapies invite a subtler discernment. They are not about peak performance or biohacking optimisation. They are about *biological belonging.* And perhaps that is the real root of malaise today—not just illness, but *estrangement.* The modern nervous system is disoriented not only by stress, but by dislocation: from place, pattern, and planet.

So the invitation is not to add more to our lives, but to subtract what occludes the essentials. Make contact with the river. Stand in the sun before checking a screen. Put bare feet to ground and notice what shifts—not just in muscle or mood, but in memory. Because these elements do not simply treat us. They *remember us.* And in that remembering, we may find a form of healing that cannot be bought, branded, or brief. Only lived.

Chapter 5
Ayurveda: The Science of Knowing Your Nature

If modern medicine speaks the language of emergencies, Ayurveda speaks the language of context. Illness, in its view, is never a random mishap but a message—a sign that the body's internal symphony has slipped out of tune. More than 5,000 years of observation, experimentation, and philosophical inquiry underpin this system, which too often is shunted into the "alternative" medicine aisle. The term does it no justice. Ayurveda is not an offshoot, nor a supplement to modern biomedicine; it is a complete lens for understanding human life—physical, emotional, ecological, and spiritual—in its constant interplay with time, place, and habit. What the wellness market has diluted is not its usefulness, but its profundity.

In the West, the most enduring distortion has been the packaging of its diagnostic vocabulary—especially the three doshas: vata, pitta, and kapha—into neat, marketable boxes. But these are not horoscope signs, nor lifestyle tribes. They are living, shifting currents of energy, perpetually altered by season, climate, diet, trauma, and age. To declare "I'm a vata" as though it were a permanent badge is to overlook Ayurveda's most disruptive insight: you are not a fixed type; you are an unfolding process. The human body is a fluid constellation of qualities, never static, always responding. The goal of Ayurveda is not to categorise you—it is to reacquaint you with your own responsiveness.

This is why the opening step in grasping Ayurveda is to discard the modern wellness tendency to flatten complex systems into quiz results and product recommendations. True understanding is not about pigeonholing but about recognising patterns. A skilled vaidya, or practitioner, doesn't stop at asking which dosha dominates; they ask how it is behaving right now—in your digestion, your dreams, your skin, your thoughts, your breath. It is this attentiveness to change that grants Ayurveda its uncanny diagnostic accuracy. It is not a static archive of facts; it is a living conversation.

At the heart of this worldview sits dinacharya—daily ritual. Not a quaint spiritual flourish, but the scaffolding that keeps the body's internal clocks in step with the wider cosmos: sunrise and sunset, waking and resting, digestion and elimination. These are not arbitrary traditions; they are the distilled wisdom of circadian alignment. Neuroscience is only now catching up to the truth Ayurveda has long held—that stability in these rhythms safeguards our brain, gut, and immune system. Disrupt them with erratic sleep, late-night screens, overstimulation, or skipped meals, and the body loses its coherence. Where a GP might diagnose anxiety, fatigue, or inflammation, Ayurveda might point to something more fundamental: a loss of rhythm.

In this light, ritual is not mere repetition. It is nervous system therapy. A glass of warm water on waking, oiling the body before a bath, eating the main meal at solar noon—these are not empty gestures. They are cues, telling the body when to wake, digest, detoxify, and slow down. Modern research confirms that such predictable sensory inputs soothe the vagus nerve, regulate cortisol, and help restore equilibrium after trauma. But Ayurveda has never needed a lab to prove what daily life already reveals: care is not a reaction—it is a rhythm.

From here, we arrive at digestion, Ayurveda's foundation stone. The term *agni*—digestive fire—goes far beyond the mechanics of enzymes and acids. It denotes the body's intelligence to transform and assimilate not only food but experience. A harsh word, an unprocessed grief, chronic sensory overload—these are also swallowed, and when not metabolised, leave behind *ama*, toxic residue. One can dine on the cleanest organic fare and yet harbour weak agni if one's relationships stifle expression, if breath never deepens, if boundaries are breached.

Contemporary science, particularly the study of the gut-brain axis, affirms much of this. But Ayurveda goes a step further: emotional digestion comes first. Eat in anger or fear, and your body will treat the food as a threat. Healing, then, is not solely about what you ingest, but about the state in which you ingest it. Treatment begins not with pills or powders but with re-establishing a sense of safety in the gut—via warmth, timing, texture, and emotional tone. Often, this means starting with *sattvic* food: uncomplicated, lightly spiced, warm meals prepared with deliberate calm. This is not romantic nostalgia; it is pure metabolic strategy.

Seen through this lens, Ayurveda's age is not a mark of obsolescence but of endurance. Its principles are not relics of a bygone culture—they are physiological constants, as relevant in today's hyper-connected, climate-controlled, overstimulated world as they were on the banks of the Saraswati. Modern patients do not usually present with a single ailment; they arrive fractured—attention frayed by devices, sleep sabotaged by artificial light, diets severed from soil, and resilience eroded by countless micro-stresses.

Ayurveda's answer is neither technophobic retreat nor rigid dogma. It does not insist on recreating the past but on restoring coherence in the present. How do we breathe deeply in the age of push notifications? How do we eat with the seasons when seasons are blurred by refrigeration? How do we protect agni when our lives run on processed speed? These are the questions for a contemporary Ayurveda that wishes to remain alive without losing its soul. The copper tongue scraper, after all, is not the cure; the awareness it cultivates is.

This chapter holds those tensions carefully, drawing on the experience of practitioners in urban clinics, trauma wards, and integrative health centres. It shares accounts of patients whose healing extended beyond better digestion or sleep to a complete reweaving of self-perception after chronic illness or identity collapse. It addresses the fine line between cultural sharing and cultural theft, the necessity of lineage respect, and the possibility of innovation without dilution.

Through it all, the through-line remains firm: Ayurveda is not a trend or a faith system. It is a science of attunement, perceiving the body as an ecosystem in constant exchange with time, space, and feeling. To know yourself is not to wear a label—it is to listen, closely and continually, to hunger and tiredness, to subtle murmurs before they become desperate shouts. Healing is less a "fix" than a homecoming, a reorientation towards clarity through the art of noticing.

This is no manual, no glossary. It is an invitation to see differently, to think more sharply, to feel more fully. In the Ayurvedic view, symptoms are not disconnected from your narrative. Your recovery will not arrive in a single capsule, but in the return of relationship—to your body, your rhythm, your sense of meaning. In a culture that craves fast solutions and frictionless ease, Ayurveda offers a rare inversion: not less thinking, but more; not rigid compliance, but subtle discernment; not external salvation, but embodied knowing. And perhaps that, in our time, is its most radical medicine.

You Are Not a Type, You Are a Tapestry

It's one of the most seductive traps in modern wellness culture: reducing the profound subtlety of an ancient medical system into a three-question quiz that declares whether you're a "Vata," "Pitta," or "Kapha" type. From lifestyle blogs to supplement labels, the doshas—cornerstones of Ayurvedic physiology—have been recast as archetypal personalities or aesthetic identities, akin to zodiac signs. But the truth is this: the doshas were never meant to label who you are. They were designed to describe what's happening within you. *To be treated according to your dosha type is a distortion. To be understood as a living, changing tapestry of qualities is Ayurvedic medicine in its true form.*

The popularisation of Ayurveda in the West has brought visibility, yes—but also flattening. Doshas, in their original context, are diagnostic principles, not static categories. Derived from Sanskrit, *Vata* governs movement, *Pitta* governs transformation, and *Kapha* governs structure and lubrication. These are not personality traits. They are *processes.* Every human being has all three in dynamic interplay, shaped by genetics, climate, emotional patterns, food, season, and age. To say someone is "a Vata" is like calling a forest a wind. *It's not wrong—it's just radically incomplete.*

A skilled Ayurvedic clinician does not begin with a dosha label. They begin with listening—*to pulse, to breath, to skin, to speech, to the story beneath the symptom.* The art lies in recognising patterns: a sharp tongue and inflamed joints might both stem from excess *Pitta,* but they may also arise from unresolved grief stored in the colon, a *Vata* site.

Diagnosis in Ayurveda is less about classification and more about *relationship*: how the elements of air, fire, water, earth, and ether express themselves uniquely in the individual. This means the same illness in two patients may be treated differently—not because their symptoms differ, but because their underlying imbalances, histories, and constitutions do.

What the Instagram version of Ayurveda misses is this *relational intelligence.* Doshas are not endpoints; they are languages. They help the practitioner trace a thread from the skin to the gut to the mind to the season to the childhood memory that keeps activating in times of stress. When we collapse this complexity into consumer-friendly boxes—"I'm Vata, so I need warm foods and slow yoga"—we lose the dynamism of Ayurvedic thinking. Worse, we externalise responsibility, waiting for the perfect dosha-aligned lifestyle to fix us, instead of cultivating internal awareness to notice when our inner climate shifts. *Dosha is not a diet plan. It's a diagnostic verb.*

This matters especially in the context of chronic stress and emotional dysregulation—the very conditions that contemporary Ayurveda is best suited to address. Because when the nervous system is frayed, the doshas misbehave. *Vata* disperses focus, causes shallow breath, and dries out digestion. *Pitta* sharpens irritability, thins patience, and overheats the gut-brain axis. *Kapha* stagnates energy, dulls mental clarity, and contributes to emotional inertia. But these are not character flaws or fixed traits. They are adaptive responses. Ayurveda recognises that the body is not malfunctioning—it's responding to overload, trying to maintain coherence with the tools it has. The goal is not to suppress the dosha, but to restore rhythm so the dosha can return to its supportive role.

Take, for example, the case of a young woman who presents with insomnia, skin inflammation, and anxiety. In a superficial reading, this could be labelled as a Pitta-Vata imbalance. But an Ayurvedic assessment would go deeper. What's her daily rhythm? When does she eat? What is the quality of her relationships? Is she waking at

2:00am because her liver is overstimulated from repressed anger? Or is she unable to sleep because her colon—ruled by Vata—is full of unprocessed grief? A dosha type is useless without context. Ayurveda always returns to *why now? Why here? Why this symptom in this body at this time?*

To honour this approach is to reclaim Ayurveda as a diagnostic philosophy rooted in observation, not prescription. This requires training—not in memorising charts or body types, but in cultivating perception. In traditional gurukula education, students spent years learning to observe pulse quality, tongue coating, eye colour, nail texture, and emotional tone before they ever offered a treatment. Today, the speed of consumer wellness demands quick identification and easy answers. But Ayurveda is not fast medicine. It is *attuned medicine*—and that attunement cannot be faked, hacked, or downloaded.

There's also an ethical dimension here. Flattening Ayurveda into typology risks not only clinical ineffectiveness but also cultural erasure. This system arose in a specific ecological and philosophical context—in dialogue with the Indian seasons, languages, food systems, and metaphysical ideas of karma, *gunas* (mental qualities), and *dhatu* (tissue development). When doshas are detached from their roots and rebranded as lifestyle aesthetics, the medicine loses its teeth. Worse, it loses its soul. *To practice or teach Ayurveda without its diagnostic subtlety is not fusion—it is fragmentation.*

And yet, Ayurveda is not rigid. It is one of the most adaptive systems of medicine ever devised. Its foundation in elemental theory makes it portable across geographies and generations. What matters is not how closely we imitate ancient routines, but how accurately we grasp *the underlying principles.* If you understand the core logic of *agni* (digestive fire), *ama* (toxins), and *guna* (qualities), you can interpret doshic imbalances in a Scandinavian winter or a Manhattan apartment. But this only works if you resist the temptation to treat doshas as identity markers. The body is not asking to be typed. It is asking to be *heard.*

We live in a time when personalisation is a marketing buzzword, yet real individualisation in medicine remains rare. Ayurveda offers a blueprint for true individual care—not by labelling patients, but by *reading their patterns over time.* This is a literacy that cannot be captured in online quizzes or simplified infographics. It must be cultivated, practiced, and—perhaps most importantly—*felt.*

This subchapter is a corrective. It is an invitation to those who have brushed up against Ayurveda and sensed its wisdom but found themselves handed a formula instead of a philosophy. It challenges even well-meaning practitioners to question where they may have collapsed nuance for clarity, or swapped diagnostic discernment for digestible content. And it encourages readers to move beyond seeking their "type" and begin asking a deeper question: *What is my system trying to tell me, in its own timing, texture, and tone?*

Because healing is not about fitting into a category. It is about reclaiming *responsiveness*—to weather, to food, to sleep, to emotion, to season, to intuition. And Ayurveda, in its truest form, doesn't label that responsiveness. It teaches you how to recognise it, live by it, and let it guide your restoration. You are not a type. You are a tapestry. And your patterns are not your prison—they are your *map.*

Ritual as Medicine

Modern life is structured by velocity—an ever-tightening spiral of productivity, distraction, and hyper-responsiveness. In this accelerated reality, routine is either dismissed as boring or weaponised as optimisation. Yet long before sleep hygiene apps and time-blocking calendars, ancient systems of medicine recognised rhythm itself as therapeutic. In Ayurveda, the daily rituals of *dinacharya* are not just wellness habits—they are treatments in their own right. These rituals anchor us to the cycles of nature and re-train our nervous system to trust predictability, stability, and pause. In a world of artificial lighting, on-demand stimulation, and chronic sympathetic overdrive, *routine is radical.* Not because it controls time—but because it restores relationship with it.

Dinacharya translates quite literally to "following the day." This is not metaphorical—it is physiological. Ayurveda posits that our bodies, like the natural world, are governed by rhythmic intelligence: the rise and fall of doshas throughout the day, the shifting elemental dominance between dawn and dusk, the hormonal orchestration of digestion, repair, and wakefulness. Rituals aligned with these cycles—waking before sunrise, cleansing the sense organs, performing self-oil massage, eating the largest meal at solar noon—are not cultural artefacts. They are neurobiological correctives. *They signal safety to a body caught in defence.*

Circadian rhythm is no longer just ancient theory—it is modern consensus. Neuroscience and chronobiology now confirm what Ayurveda has long observed: the timing of behaviours has a profound effect on gene expression, immunity, metabolism, and cognitive clarity. A study published in *Cell* (2017) showed that over 40% of human genes are under circadian control. When these rhythms are disrupted by erratic schedules, late-night light exposure, or irregular eating, systems fall out of coherence. The nervous system becomes less resilient, inflammation rises, and recovery falters. But when rituals are introduced that stabilise timing—rising and sleeping at consistent hours, taking food when digestive fire is naturally strongest—physiology begins to reorganise. What feels "subtle" in practice is actually biologically significant.

More than time-bound habits, dinacharya is a form of somatic re-education. Its power lies not just in what is done, but in how it is done. For instance, *abhyanga*—the practice of daily warm oil self-massage—is far more than moisturising. It is an embodied language. The slow, rhythmic strokes down the limbs and across the chest stimulate lymphatic drainage, reduce cortisol, and trigger vagal tone. But perhaps more importantly, *they remind the body it is safe to inhabit itself.* For those recovering from trauma, stress, or burnout, this ritual can be a turning point: an act of reconnection that doesn't require language, only touch.

This somatic effect is not incidental. Ayurveda understands that trauma and chronic stress erode the *ojas*—the subtle essence of immunity, vitality, and emotional buoyancy. Rebuilding ojas is not accomplished through effort. It is cultivated through rituals that restore containment and cohesion. Consistency, slowness, gentleness—these qualities form the architecture of ojas. And while supplements may support it, *no capsule can replace the nervous system's need for predictability.* Daily rituals, practiced with presence and care, re-pattern that predictability into the tissues.

Consider the ritual of mindful elimination upon waking—a seemingly mundane task that Ayurveda elevates to sacred timing. The colon is the seat of *Vata*, the dosha most implicated in stress-related conditions: anxiety, insomnia, bloating, dissociation. By emptying the bowels in the early morning, when Vata is naturally dominant, we clear not only waste but also emotional residue. Paired with warm water, tongue scraping, and nasal oiling, this routine becomes a subtle but potent morning detox—not just of the gut, but of mental clutter. The cumulative effect over weeks and months is a body that begins the day with clarity, not chaos.

Western clinical research is beginning to catch up. Studies in behavioural neuroscience indicate that consistent morning routines reduce cortisol variability and improve emotional regulation. A paper in *Frontiers in Psychology* (2019) linked ritualistic behaviours with lower anxiety and greater resilience, particularly in high-stress environments. Yet what these studies often overlook is the *symbolic intelligence* of ritual. Dinacharya doesn't just work because it optimises function—it works because it reinstates meaning. It reminds the person that life is not random, that there is a rhythm to belong to.

And this matters deeply in our time. Mental health is not only about neurotransmitters. It is also about disconnection—*from body, from time, from place, from purpose.* Dinacharya gently mends those severed links. It says: there is a time to rise, to cleanse, to eat, to rest. Not because discipline is moral, but because the body is rhythmic by design. The nervous system, battered by the noise and novelty of modernity, craves not more stimulation but more *sequence.* When we wake at the same hour, eat in calm, tend our senses with intention, and rest in rhythm with the dark, we begin to hear the body's original song. Ritual is not a restriction. It is a restoration of belonging.

Still, to be effective, rituals must be relational, not robotic. Performing dinacharya as a checklist undermines its healing intelligence. The aim is not to perfect every detail but to cultivate intimacy with timing. A mother rising early to boil tea before the house wakes, a commuter placing a drop of rose oil in the nostrils before entering the subway, a student closing the laptop at sundown and lighting a lamp—*these are not performances.* They are micro-acts of nervous system repair, nested in the reality of daily life. When approached this way, ritual becomes not another item on the to-do list, but a *way of being in time that fosters coherence.*

This brings us to a critical point: *ritual is different from routine.* Routine is often externally imposed, oriented toward productivity or control. Ritual, in contrast, is imbued with *presence, pattern, and purpose.* It is less about what you do and more about the intention behind it. In Ayurveda, brushing the teeth is not hygiene alone—it is a cleansing of the morning breath to clear the voice. Applying oil to the scalp is not grooming—it is calming the prefrontal cortex, where stress hijacks focus. Every act, however small, becomes an opportunity to remind the body of its place in the living cosmos.

For practitioners working with clients recovering from burnout, insomnia, hormonal imbalances, or chronic fatigue, introducing ritual can be more impactful than prescribing supplements or diet changes. Start with rhythm. One regular wake time. One consistent sleep cue. One mindful breath before meals. These are not trivial gestures. They are the scaffolding of recovery. Because the body's repair mechanisms do not thrive on novelty—they thrive on *trust.* And trust is built through rhythm.

This is the deep lesson of dinacharya: *rituals repair what stress disorders.* They are not cosmetic, exotic, or archaic. They are medicine—encoded in the logic of the body, and echoed by millennia of lived wisdom. They may look humble from the outside, but practiced with care, they hold the power to recalibrate systems far beneath the surface. In a hyperactive world, where complexity is often confused with sophistication, *returning to rhythm is an act of both healing and resistance.*

Ritual does not require wealth, equipment, or time abundance. It asks only that we honour timing, attention, and simplicity. This is a paradigm shift. It challenges the assumption that healing must be hard or expensive. Dinacharya shows that what the body often needs most is not more—but *again.* Again the same breath. Again the same gesture. Again the same rising sun. Repetition is not stagnation—it is recalibration. And in that rhythm, the nervous system exhales, the mind softens, and the body begins to remember how to be whole.

Digestion as the Gateway to Emotional and Energetic Health

In modern biomedicine, digestion is often reduced to a mechanical process—enzymes breaking down food, nutrients absorbed, waste expelled. But in Ayurveda, digestion is not merely what happens in the gut. It is *the primary axis of health,* determining the clarity of our thoughts, the sharpness of our memory, the quality of our energy, and the resilience of our emotions. The Sanskrit term *agni*—meaning fire—is the cornerstone of this understanding. Agni is more than just stomach acid or metabolic rate. It is the intelligent fire that governs transformation in every cell, sense, and subtle channel of the body. And when that fire is disrupted, by stress, trauma, or habitual dysregulation, the disturbance doesn't stop in the intestines. *It spreads systemically—clouding the mind, weakening the heart, and dulling the will to act.*

Ayurveda identifies multiple levels of agni—from the central digestive fire in the gut (*jatharagni*), to the tissue-specific fires (*dhatu agni*), to the cellular fires responsible for vitality and repair. These flames must be balanced—not too weak, not too fierce—for life to function harmoniously. Weak agni leads to *ama*, a Sanskrit term for undigested residue, often described as metabolic sludge. Ama is not just physical; it is emotional and cognitive too. Unprocessed grief, repressed anger, chronic indecision—these too are forms of undigested experience, sticking in the system like half-cooked food. In this way, *impaired digestion becomes both cause and symptom of deeper imbalance.*

Clinical Ayurvedic practitioners routinely observe the correlation between digestive dysfunction and mental health. Consider a patient presenting with bloating, brain fog, poor appetite, and episodic depression. From a biomedical perspective, these might seem like unrelated issues, treated by separate specialists. But in Ayurvedic practice, they often stem from the same root: disturbed agni. Without sufficient fire, food stagnates, toxins accumulate, and the mind loses its clarity. Restoring agni—through dietary rhythm, herbal support, emotional processing, and lifestyle alignment—becomes a unifying treatment that reclaims both digestive and emotional coherence.

This is not speculative. Contemporary psychogastroenterology, a field emerging at the intersection of gut and mental health, now affirms what Ayurveda has long known: *the gut is not only the site of digestion, but a central command post for mood regulation, trauma recovery, and cognitive performance.* More than 90% of serotonin receptors are located in the gastrointestinal tract. The vagus nerve, the primary channel of parasympathetic regulation, sends more signals from gut to brain than the other way around. Chronic stress leads to gut inflammation; gut inflammation heightens anxiety and depressive symptoms. This feedback loop is not merely chemical—it is energetic and emotional.

Ayurveda, however, adds a crucial layer of understanding: not all digestive issues stem from diet. Often, they stem from *emotional indigestion.* A client may be eating all the right foods, yet still experiencing reflux or constipation because they are holding unresolved grief in the chest, or suppressed rage in the liver. One practitioner described a patient who suffered years of IBS-like symptoms, unresponsive to elimination diets. Through Ayurvedic assessment and *manovaha srota* (mind-body channel) analysis, it was revealed that the digestive fire was erratic because the patient was repressing long-standing shame around a broken family relationship. With therapeutic support, the use of grounding herbs like *ashwagandha* and *vidari*, and the introduction of mindful eating rituals that included gratitude and intentional chewing, symptoms subsided—not because of restriction, but because of *integration.*

This relational approach to digestion reframes treatment from exclusion to assimilation. The aim is not merely to eliminate triggers, but to *strengthen the system's capacity to digest life itself.* This includes food, yes, but also emotion, sensory input, and interpersonal experience. Agni, in this light, is a measure of one's ability to metabolise reality. And the gut is not only a biomechanical engine—it is a site of discernment. To digest well is to discern wisely—what to absorb, what to eliminate, what to transform.

Daily practices can reinforce this discernment. Eating with full attention—not in front of screens or amidst multitasking—activates the cephalic phase of digestion and supports parasympathetic tone. Using herbs like *trikatu* (a blend of black pepper, long pepper, and ginger) stokes agni gently without overdriving it. Respecting the body's call for hunger, rather than eating by the clock, retrains digestive intelligence. These may seem like small acts, but in aggregate, they retrain the nervous system toward coherence. Ayurveda teaches that *agni is not stoked by willpower—it is nourished by rhythm.*

Trauma complicates this rhythm. Many trauma survivors experience a chronic disconnection from hunger cues, disrupted bowel patterns, and erratic eating habits. The gut becomes both hypersensitive and hypo-responsive. For these individuals, rebuilding digestive strength is not a matter of diet alone—it is a process of *re-establishing safety in the body*. This is where the use of gentle digestive rituals—like sipping warm cumin-coriander-fennel tea, applying warm castor oil packs over the abdomen, or simply pausing to breathe before meals—can be therapeutic. These practices signal to the enteric nervous system that it is safe to digest, safe to receive, and safe to let go.

Notably, agni is not static. It changes throughout the day, the seasons, and the life cycle. Ayurveda teaches that *agni is strongest at midday*, when the sun is highest, and weakest after sunset, when cooling, lunar energies dominate. Eating the main meal at midday supports digestive efficiency and mental clarity. Similarly, agni tends to weaken during the cold, damp seasons, requiring warming spices and cooked foods, while in the summer, lighter fare aligns with the already heightened internal heat. By aligning our eating with these cycles, we support agni's natural fluctuations instead of working against them.

This cyclical understanding challenges the modern tendency to impose one-size-fits-all dietary prescriptions. What nourishes one person may burden another. Two individuals with similar symptoms may have entirely different agni types—one with a sharp, overactive fire leading to hyperacidity and anger; the other with a low, flickering flame that struggles to digest even simple meals, often coupled with sadness or fatigue. The key is not what diet is universally best, but what supports *your* agni in this season of life. This diagnostic subtlety is what elevates Ayurveda from a system of rules to a system of *relationship*.

Energetically, digestion is more than nourishment—it is purification. Agni, when balanced, transforms both food and experience into *ojas*, the subtle essence that gives radiance to the skin, depth to sleep, compassion to the heart, and steadiness to the mind. When agni is impaired, the result is *ama*, which clouds the mind, dulls the senses, and blocks emotional flow. Thus, the quality of digestion sets the tone for how a person engages with life—whether they move from clarity or confusion, responsiveness or reactivity.

In a society increasingly dominated by mental fog, mood instability, and metabolic disorder, the Ayurvedic view of digestion offers a profound reorientation. It teaches us that the path to mental clarity is not always cognitive. Often, it begins in the gut—with warm food, consistent meals, and emotional safety. It challenges the overemphasis on control—of calories, macronutrients, or willpower—and replaces it with an emphasis on *trust*: trust in rhythm, in the body's wisdom, and in the healing fire within.

Agni is not merely a metaphor. It is a biological and spiritual compass. When it is clear, we are clear. When it is erratic, we are unstable. When it is extinguished, we are unwell. The restoration of agni is not about returning to some ideal digestive state. It is about cultivating the conditions for intelligent transformation—*digesting what is ours to keep, releasing what must pass, and building the vitality to meet life with steadiness*. This is the work of digestion. And it is the foundation of emotional and energetic health.

Ayurveda in the Anthropocene

Ayurveda emerged not from abstraction but from direct, sustained intimacy with the natural world. Its diagnostic and therapeutic frameworks were formed through careful observation of ecological rhythms—of sunlight and moonlight, seasons and soil, hunger and rest. The Rishis, Ayurveda's seers, did not merely theorise health; they *lived inside the patterns* that governed it. But today, we no longer live within those same patterns. The Anthropocene—our current epoch defined by human-driven planetary disruption—poses profound challenges to this lineage. Climate instability, ecological collapse, chronic overstimulation, urban alienation, and a globalised mental health crisis raise a critical question: *Can an ancient system like Ayurveda remain relevant in an age it never anticipated?*

The short answer is yes—but only if we engage with it as a living philosophy, not a static tradition. To do so requires us to differentiate between Ayurveda's *form* and its *function*. The form—the herbs, rituals, seasonal diets—arose from a specific bioregional context: subcontinental India, with its monsoons, agrarian economy, and close-knit village life. But the function—the principles of *rhythm, relationship, regulation, and right discernment*—is universal and adaptive. When we abstract these principles from their historical packaging, we gain the tools to address the pathologies of modern life without diluting Ayurveda's essence.

Climate change is not only a planetary crisis; it is a constitutional one. Ayurveda teaches that balance arises from harmony between the internal and external environment. When seasons are stable, agni—the digestive fire—tends to be steady. When days and nights are predictable, sleep and metabolism regulate naturally. But the Anthropocene is marked by disordered seasons, artificial light cycles, disrupted food webs, and increasing climatic volatility. The body registers this. What we see clinically is an epidemic of vata-aggravation: dry skin, constipation, insomnia, anxiety, and overwhelm. The vata dosha—linked to air and ether—is especially sensitive to speed, unpredictability, and disconnection. These are not merely personal ailments; they are *ecological symptoms* expressed through the human organism.

In this context, Ayurveda's seasonal routines (*ritucharya*) become not just health advice but *acts of resistance*. When we align our sleep, food, and activity to solar and lunar rhythms—eating with daylight, resting after sunset, adjusting our routines with the seasons—we reclaim autonomy from an economy that profits from our disorientation. For example, in the dead of winter, modern life asks for constant productivity under LED lights. Ayurveda counsels warm, cooked meals, slower mornings, and inward attention. These are not indulgences; they are metabolic necessities. If the outside world no longer cues our biology reliably, the onus falls on us to recreate that rhythm intentionally. *Dinacharya*—the daily rituals of waking, cleansing, oiling, eating, and resting—becomes the scaffolding that restores nervous system integrity in a time of unrelenting flux.

Technology, while amplifying access to Ayurvedic knowledge, also poses new stressors to the very systems Ayurveda seeks to balance. Excess screen time distorts the circadian cycle. Notifications hijack attention. Algorithmic feeds overstimulate the sensory channels (*indriyas*), diluting the mind's digestive fire (*manas agni*). The cumulative effect is fragmentation—not only of focus, but of selfhood. One loses touch with *pratyahara*, the Ayurvedic principle of inward sensory withdrawal necessary for discernment and integration. For many patients today, the first step in Ayurvedic healing is not a new herb or recipe, but *a confrontation with technological overexposure*.

Some contemporary practitioners have adapted classical protocols to address this. For example, digital fasting—unplugging from screens at least one hour before bed—is now prescribed alongside *triphala* for gut repair. The logic is coherent: the gut and brain are connected via the vagus nerve, and overstimulated senses disrupt this bi-directional communication. Similarly, modern *panchakarma* centres increasingly integrate digital detox with traditional oil therapies, recognising that restoration of *ojas*—our vital essence—requires not only physical purification but energetic withdrawal from information pollution. These innovations do not betray Ayurveda's roots; they extend its logic into present-day terrain.

Mental health, perhaps more than any other domain, illustrates both the urgency and potential of Ayurvedic application in the Anthropocene. The World Health Organization now cites depression as the leading cause of disability worldwide. Anxiety, burnout, and trauma-related disorders are rampant. Standard pharmacological treatments offer partial relief but often fail to address the *systemic and existential dimensions* of suffering. Ayurveda approaches the psyche not as separate from the soma, but as an energetic continuum. The mind (*manas*) is not housed in the brain alone—it circulates through every tissue, shaped by food, breath, thought, and environment. Therefore, mental distress is rarely treated in isolation. A patient with panic attacks may receive *brahmi* and *shankhpushpi* for the mind, but also *ghee* to stabilise vata, *nasya* oil for the sinuses, and morning sun exposure to reset melatonin-cortisol rhythms.

Where modern psychiatry pathologises symptoms, Ayurveda contextualises them. A woman presenting with anxiety, cold extremities, and dry skin is not simply given a DSM diagnosis; she is understood as having *vata vriddhi*, possibly exacerbated by overwork, travel, erratic meals, and emotional loss. Treatment becomes a layered process: grounding foods, stable routine, warm oil massage (*abhyanga*), and emotionally attuned dialogue. This holistic model acknowledges what the Anthropocene so often obscures: that *well-being is relational, rhythmic, and ecologically situated.* To feel safe in one's body requires feeling safe in one's environment—and today, neither can be taken for granted.

Even the globalisation of Ayurveda itself must be interrogated within this frame. As the wellness industry grows, Ayurvedic herbs are commodified, exported, and packaged in ways that sometimes ignore their ecological footprint. The mass harvesting of *ashwagandha* or *turmeric* for Western markets raises ethical questions: can we promote sustainability and sacredness simultaneously? Some herbalists and physicians are now advocating for *bioregional Ayurveda*—the application of Ayurvedic principles using local plants, foods, and practices. This not only reduces environmental strain, but restores Ayurveda's original orientation: *contextual medicine rooted in place.*

Adaptation also means decolonisation. For centuries, Ayurveda was suppressed under colonial regimes that deemed indigenous knowledge inferior to Western science. Today, that suppression often re-emerges in subtler forms—through appropriation, oversimplification, or tokenised inclusion. Reclaiming Ayurveda's full depth involves restoring its philosophical underpinnings: *sankhya*, *guna*, *karma*, *dharma*—the cosmological frameworks that give it coherence. It also involves amplifying voices from within Ayurvedic lineages—practitioners, scholars, and elders who carry lived understanding that cannot be downloaded or credentialed.

Crucially, Ayurveda in the Anthropocene cannot afford to be nostalgic. While its roots are ancient, its relevance depends on its *responsiveness*. Climate grief, ecological anxiety, and techno-spiritual burnout are real afflictions. Ayurveda must meet them not with platitudes, but with *precision*. For the practitioner, this means studying not only Sanskrit and srotas, but also trauma theory, climate science, and systems thinking. It means seeing dosha not as typecasting, but as dynamic patterns affected by everything from urban design to economic inequality. It means recognising that healing is not only individual, but collective and planetary.

This expansion does not weaken Ayurveda; it fulfils it. At its core, Ayurveda is a science of balance—between body and world, self and other, consumption and conservation. The Anthropocene is a time of imbalance, of exceeding limits, of forgetting interdependence. Ayurveda offers not only tools for symptom relief, but a *philosophical recalibration*: that to live well is to live in right relation. This is its medicine. And in this epoch of disruption, it is medicine we urgently need.

Chapter 6
Energy Without Stimulants: Eastern Therapies for Flow and Vitality

Exhaustion, for many, has slipped quietly from being an occasional state into the unspoken baseline of modern life. Even with our supposed abundance of time-saving devices and a buffet of productivity tools, few genuinely feel alive in the marrow-deep sense of the word. What we tend to call "energy" is often little more than a jittery scaffolding—propped up by caffeine, fuelled by urgency, sustained by distraction. The nervous system, overstimulated yet strangely starved, borrows from tomorrow to function today. It runs on adrenal debt rather than the quiet reserves of natural rhythm. Against this restless backdrop, Eastern energy medicine stands apart—not as another means of revving the engine, but as an entirely different current. Not hype, but harmony. Not effort, but flow.

In the lexicon of Eastern traditions—qi in Chinese medicine, prana in Ayurveda—energy is no metaphor, nor merely a tally of calories consumed. It is the very substance of life, felt and moved through specific channels (meridians or nadis), responsive to posture, breath, intention, and attention. Within these systems, vitality isn't manufactured through force; it's uncovered, tended to, and allowed to circulate. Often it's not absent at all—merely blocked, scattered, or leaking away. Thus, energy medicine is not so much a skill to master as it is a stance to inhabit, a way of perceiving one's own internal weather.

Here, we approach subtle energy with both a clinician's grounding and a contemplative eye. First, qi and prana will be introduced not as exotic terms to memorise, but as realities one can encounter directly. Through stories from both patients and practitioners, we will trace how these currents are sensed, mapped, and restored. A burnt-out corporate leader, for example, learns to recognise the hollow, caffeinated buzz that once passed for energy, and to distinguish it from the steadier undercurrent of balanced qi—measured not in output, but in digestion, breath, and unbroken sleep. The question is never "do you believe in prana?" but "can you feel the difference when you are agitated, rested, angry, or quietly still?"

From this understanding, we move into the practical territory of acupressure. Unlike acupuncture, which calls for years of specialised training, acupressure is immediate, non-invasive, and unexpectedly self-empowering. A nurse with evening panic episodes learns to steady herself by pressing Heart 7 (Shenmen); a student with a restless stomach works with Stomach 36 (Zusanli) before meals to restore balance. These points are not magic switches—they are portals into a conversation the body has been trying to hold all along, reconnecting organs, emotions, and awareness into a more harmonious dialogue.

What underpins these methods is a distinct ethic about where power lies. Western notions of energy often veer toward extraction—do more, rest less, optimise endlessly. Eastern therapies, in contrast, invite a more relational question: what happens if you do less, but do it with full presence? This dovetails with the Taoist principle of *wu wei*—commonly mistaken for passivity, but in truth the refined art of action arising without strain. The Taoist butcher, whose blade never dulls because he moves with the grain of the meat, exemplifies this. Neurologically, this is the body returning to a state where the parasympathetic system—nature's own restorer—can quietly do its work.

Nor is this mode of living confined to stillness. It threads through movement forms that listen before they lead—Qi Gong, tai chi, breath-oriented yoga, mindful walking. A retired engineer with high blood pressure takes up Qi Gong, not to "work out" but to fine-tune his perception. Over time, he notices the subtle recalibrations: a softened posture, shifting cravings, a longer patience. Fatigue is no longer something to outpace; energy has become a tide to move with.

Such examples are becoming less anecdotal and more emblematic of a quiet rebellion against the stimulant economy—an economy that mistakes activation for vitality, speed for direction. Eastern energy traditions counter with different measures: not how long you can maintain output, but how completely you can replenish; not the sharpness of focus, but the spaciousness of attention.

Crucially, these systems don't simply sit beside Western medicine as optional extras; they question its foundations. Where biomedicine often sees the body as a passive mechanism, acted upon by chemical interventions, energy medicine sees a responsive, patterned field. A person with chronic fatigue may receive "normal" blood test results and a prescription for antidepressants, while an energy-based approach might find sluggishness in the liver meridian, unresolved grief lodged in the lungs, or cold stagnation in the lower abdomen. Treatment becomes an invitation rather than a suppression—breath into frozen places, warmth into cold tissues, rhythm into a scattered existence.

This reframing matters most in the context of stress disorders that are now near-ubiquitous among the high-functioning. A fortnightly yoga class or a dash of herbal supplementation will not reverse sympathetic overdrive. What's needed is a rethinking of the very metaphor we use: are you a battery to be charged and drained, or an ecosystem to be nourished and tended? The former leads to temporary highs and eventual collapse; the latter, to sustainable vitality and a more rooted sense of self.

Throughout these pages, our purpose is not to reduce these ideas into yet another checklist for "optimisation," but to open a more porous doorway into relationship with life force itself. Small, consistent gestures—an acupressure point pressed with intention, a breath followed to its quiet end, a jaw released from its clench—can, when given attention, become agents of profound change. Vitality ceases to be a commodity to seek elsewhere; it becomes an inner climate you can tend directly.

The people who carry these traditions forward—acupuncturists working with trauma survivors, Qi Gong teachers guiding elders, poets capturing stillness in words—remind us of one thing: real energy does not arrive through force. It returns when we've learned to listen for it.

That is the quiet challenge of this work: not to strive harder, nor to accumulate techniques, but to refine your listening. To know the difference between adrenaline and genuine presence, between pushing and moving in alignment, between depletion and the deep current of flow. Energy without stimulants is not a utopian idea—it is among the most ancient medicines we have, requiring no pills, no purchases, no performance. Only the willingness to pay attention, and the trust to let the body remember what it already knows.

Qi and Prana: The Hidden Currents of Health

Most people can sense when their energy is "off"—a vague heaviness in the limbs, a restless mind that won't quiet, or a disconnection from the day's rhythm. Yet in modern biomedicine, this lived experience of vitality has no formal category. Fatigue might be noted, stress acknowledged, but rarely is the language of subtle energy considered valid. Traditional systems like Chinese medicine and Ayurveda take the opposite approach: they begin with energy. *Qi* and *prana* are not abstract metaphors or cultural superstitions—they are diagnostic tools, therapeutic maps, and most critically, experiential truths. To ignore them is not scientific humility; it is a narrowing of perception that costs us resilience, clarity, and healing.

Qi (氣), in classical Chinese thought, is the animating force of life. It is what distinguishes a corpse from a living being. Not simply breath, nor merely electrical impulse, it is a field of dynamic intelligence—circulating through meridians, concentrating in organs, and influenced by everything from food and sleep to emotions and relationships. Prana, the Sanskrit analogue, is similarly multidimensional. It flows through the nadis (energy channels) and governs both gross physiological processes (like respiration) and subtler states of awareness. These concepts are not interchangeable, but they are analogous in one critical respect: *they assert that health is not just chemical or mechanical, but energetic.* When energy flows smoothly, vitality follows. When it stagnates, dissipates, or becomes erratic, dysfunction arises.

To appreciate the value of these models, one must shift from passive observation to embodied sensing. In practice, this means learning to feel energy—not as a metaphorical idea, but as a concrete internal current. Consider the common experience of holding the breath in stress, of feeling heat rise during anger, or of sensing a "gut feeling" that precedes conscious thought. These are not poetic flourishes; they are expressions of energetic activity. A trauma survivor may notice a tightness in the chest that no CT scan explains, yet a skilled acupuncturist or Ayurvedic practitioner might immediately identify blocked heart qi or disturbed prana vayu. *The symptom is not just in the tissue—it is in the current that feeds it.*

Stress, in both traditions, is primarily understood not in terms of cortisol or adrenaline, but in terms of flow. Chronic worry scatters qi, leaving the mind fragmented and the body depleted. Grief contracts the lung qi, resulting in shallow breath and suppressed immunity. Excessive multitasking disperses prana, creating mental fog, digestive instability, and emotional volatility. These descriptions do not negate neurochemical explanations; they expand them. Rather than pathologising each symptom in isolation, energy medicine invites us to *trace the pattern that connects them*, and to restore coherence through subtle regulation.

Regulation, in this context, does not mean suppression. It means restoring rhythm and responsiveness. Breath is the most immediate access point. Both qi and prana are intimately tied to respiration—not just in mechanics, but in quality. Shallow, erratic breathing reflects a dysregulated energetic state. Slow, deep, rhythmic breathing generates coherence across physiological and subtle systems. A practitioner of Qi Gong may begin their morning by cultivating *dan tian* energy through soft abdominal breath. An Ayurvedic clinician might teach *nadi shodhana* (alternate nostril breathing) to balance pranic flow between the left and right channels. These are not spiritual practices in the reductive sense—they are *interventions in energetic architecture.*

The concept of energy regulation also invites ethical reflection. In Western paradigms, energy is something to be managed, boosted, or optimised. In Eastern systems, energy is something to be respected. Overexertion, overexposure, and overconsumption are seen as violations—not of a moral code, but of a natural law. For example, staying up late against one's circadian rhythm is not just poor sleep hygiene—it is an assault on the descending movement of prana that governs rest and repair. Similarly, excessive talking or stimulation may scatter qi, leaving the practitioner depleted not because they "did too much," but because they *acted out of rhythm with their own flow.*

Real-world applications of energy literacy are increasingly being documented. In integrative oncology clinics, acupuncture is used not simply to treat pain, but to support vitality during chemotherapy by stabilising spleen and kidney qi. In trauma therapy settings, somatic experiencing practitioners draw upon the principles of grounded presence—akin to centred prana—to help clients titrate difficult emotions. In advanced yoga therapy, subtle body assessments guide the sequencing of breath, posture, and attention in ways that move blocked energy without overwhelming the nervous system. These are not fringe ideas—they are part of a growing paradigm shift that recognises the body as a field of communication, not a battleground of symptoms.

Importantly, learning to sense energy is not a mystical skill reserved for the initiated. It is a human birthright, long suppressed by intellectual overreach and sensory disconnection. Children know it intuitively. They contract around conflict, brighten with harmony, and regulate through rhythmic play. Adults can relearn this, but only through *direct experience.* No amount of reading about qi will substitute for the moment when you feel it—palpably, undeniably—moving through your spine in meditation, or settling your gut after breath-led relaxation. That moment shifts energy from theory to reality.

This capacity to sense energy is not merely self-indulgent—it is foundational to resilience. A person who can track their energetic state is less likely to override signals of burnout. They will notice early tremors of depletion, honour the need for rest, and adjust their pace accordingly. This is what energy medicine calls *living in right rhythm.* It is not always convenient, but it is always intelligent. In times of chronic stress and ecological breakdown, the ability to sense and regulate internal flow becomes not a luxury but a necessity.

Yet, there is an inevitable tension between these systems and the demands of modern life. How can one live in harmony with qi or prana while working 60-hour weeks under artificial lighting and digital overload? This question is not rhetorical. It is the challenge of our era. The answer is not withdrawal, but *strategic recalibration.* Even amidst structural pressures, micro-practices can restore flow. Five minutes of coherent breathing between meetings. Acupressure on Liver 3 during irritability. A barefoot walk on soil to discharge stagnant energy. These are not aesthetic gestures; they are *acts of recalibration* in an otherwise dysrhythmic world.

Understanding qi and prana also requires intellectual humility. These frameworks do not pretend to explain everything, but they do point to dimensions of experience that biomedicine routinely neglects. Rather than pit one model against the other, a more mature approach is integrative pluralism: using energy models to interpret meaning, biomedical models to measure mechanics, and always letting the patient's felt experience guide the way. When a clinician asks not just "Where does it hurt?" but "Where does the energy feel stuck?" they are not abandoning science—they are *widening the lens of inquiry.*

The promise of energy literacy is not that we will feel euphoric all the time. It is that we will *become intelligent stewards of our own flow.* We will begin to notice how certain environments deplete us while others replenish us. We will stop measuring vitality in terms of hours worked or goals achieved, and start recognising it in how well we digest, sleep, and relate. We will learn that real energy does not shout—it hums. It whispers. It pulses. And it can be restored not through stimulation, but through alignment.

That is the true medicine of qi and prana: not a supplement or shortcut, but a return to coherence. A way of living in which the body is not a machine to be driven, but a current to be followed. A way of seeing in which stress is not the enemy, but a signal—an invitation to feel more deeply, respond more wisely, and restore what was never lost, only forgotten.

Acupressure and Meridian Alchemy

There is a growing fatigue with overcomplication in modern health discourse. Many are exhausted not just by their symptoms, but by the machinery surrounding their management—overmedicalisation, overmedication, and the constant deferral to specialists. Against this backdrop, the re-emergence of hands-on, non-invasive modalities like acupressure signals more than a revival of ancient techniques. It suggests a return to intelligibility. Acupressure offers not just symptom relief but *somatic literacy*—a means of communicating with the body through touch, pattern, and presence.

Unlike acupuncture, which requires needles and formal training, acupressure is accessible. With nothing more than informed fingers and attentive awareness, individuals can begin to influence their internal states by stimulating specific points—*gateways in the body's energetic network*. These are not arbitrary zones but deeply mapped locations on meridians, the invisible yet palpable lines through which qi flows. When properly activated, these points do more than relieve pain or tension; they recalibrate systems, modulate emotions, and re-establish rhythm where stress has disrupted flow.

For many, the first experience of acupressure is not profound, but instructive. A light pressure at the base of the skull during a headache, a firm press on the centre of the palm during a moment of panic. The effects may be subtle—a slowing of the breath, a softening of the jaw—but they signal a shift from passive distress to active agency. Practitioners often describe this not as treatment, but as *dialogue* between hand and meridian, between surface and core.

One widely used point for nervous system regulation is Pericardium 6, or Neiguan. Located three finger-widths below the wrist crease, between the two tendons in the forearm, this point is known to settle the heart-mind connection. In Chinese medicine, the pericardium is more than an anatomical sac; it is an emotional shield, protecting the heart from sudden shocks and chronic overstimulation. When activated through sustained pressure, Neiguan can reduce anxiety, soothe nausea (especially when linked to stress), and help regulate a hyperaroused vagus nerve. Patients in integrative cardiology clinics have reported reduced palpitations and panic symptoms after learning to self-stimulate this point in high-stress moments.

Another crucial point is Kidney 1, Yongquan, found on the sole of the foot. In Taoist medicine, this is where the body's energy enters from the earth. It is often used to ground scattered or erratic qi—especially in individuals experiencing insomnia, dissociation, or chronic overthinking. In clinical settings, acupressure here is used to "draw down" excessive activity from the head, allowing the nervous system to reorient toward stillness. This isn't relaxation as sedation, but as *repatterning*: a way to reset the feedback loop between the central nervous system and the body's deeper currents.

Real-world examples illustrate this more vividly than theory alone. A trauma therapist in Vancouver incorporates acupressure into her somatic sessions, teaching clients to press Spleen 6 (located on the inner leg, just above the ankle) while engaging in gentle guided breathing. The point is known to stabilise the lower burner—the part of the body most reactive to fear, urgency, and adrenal fatigue. One client, a war veteran with PTSD, reported that learning to hold this point while grounding visually in his environment allowed him, for the first time in years, to *interrupt the freeze response before it escalated into a panic attack*. The technique didn't cure him, but it gave him access to regulation, which no pharmaceutical had managed to do alone.

Critics of energy-based modalities often ask: where is the evidence? The challenge is that much of the efficacy of acupressure resists reduction into isolated variables. Clinical trials are emerging, showing effects on heart rate variability, cortisol levels, and sleep quality. But to truly grasp the value of meridian alchemy, one must experience the layered nature of healing it enables. A patient may arrive with chronic fatigue and insomnia and leave not just with more energy, but with an intuitive sense of what their body is asking for. This is *biofeedback without machinery*, requiring only the will to feel and the discipline to listen.

The language of meridians often deters modern readers, sounding esoteric or outdated. But when reframed as functional circuits—maps of interoceptive intelligence—they begin to resemble systems science more than superstition. For example, the Liver meridian, which governs the smooth flow of qi and emotional regulation, often becomes congested in individuals with chronic irritability, menstrual irregularities, or tension headaches. Pressing Liver 3 (between the big toe and second toe) regularly can "move stuckness" not only physiologically but psychospiritually. Patients often report improved clarity, reduced emotional volatility, and less somatic tension. *The body speaks in patterns; meridians provide the grammar.*

Practitioners often describe the meridian system as fractal and holographic: every part reflects the whole. This is why certain points—such as Large Intestine 4 on the hand—can influence the head and face, while Gallbladder 21 on the shoulder can relieve tension in the pelvis. This cross-talk may seem improbable until one considers the fascial and neurological continuities that modern anatomy is only beginning to map. In this way, acupressure becomes a bridge—not only across systems of the body, but across paradigms of knowledge.

Importantly, acupressure is not a mechanical task. It requires attunement. Pressure that is too hard can agitate the nervous system; too soft, and it may not penetrate the deeper energetic layer. The practitioner must learn to *feel for receptivity*, adjusting not only their fingers but their state of presence. A distracted touch yields little; a connected one transforms. This is why seasoned practitioners often teach patients to pair point stimulation with breath, awareness, and even sound. The point becomes an access node—not a magic button, but a threshold for integrated healing.

There is also a cultural humility needed when borrowing these practices. Acupressure is rooted in centuries of Taoist and Confucian medical philosophy. To extract points from their context—reducing them to "hacks" for stress—risks stripping them of their coherence. True engagement means learning not only where the points are, but *why they matter within the larger cosmology of health.* This means recognising that the meridian system reflects not just anatomy, but ethics: balance, reciprocity, seasonality, and restraint.

Modern life works against these principles. The pace is erratic, the stimuli overwhelming, the disconnection from body nearly total. Acupressure, in this context, becomes a radical act—not because it is exotic, but because it reintroduces something ancient and sane. A practitioner pressing a point is not merely fixing a dysfunction; they are reawakening a relationship. The body is not an object to be manipulated but a field to be harmonised.

For beginners, the path is not to memorise every point, but to start with a few and observe. Try Pericardium 6 before bed. Explore Liver 3 during midday agitation. Hold Kidney 1 while lying in the grass. Track not just the sensation, but the ripple effect—what changes in breath, thought, emotion. Then repeat, not as a technique, but as a form of listening. Over time, patterns will emerge, and the body will begin to respond with a clarity that no app or device can offer.

In a world hungry for agency yet saturated with distraction, acupressure offers something rare: *an intelligent simplicity.* With nothing more than time-tested maps and one's own hands, it invites a direct engagement with the nervous system—not through control, but through co-regulation. It is not a panacea, nor a replacement for allopathic care. But it is a powerful complement—restoring not just the balance of systems, but the dignity of self-healing.

The Tao of Doing Less

There is an unspoken violence embedded in our modern metrics of success. The compulsion to produce, accelerate, optimise, and outperform has infiltrated not only our workplaces, but our minds and bodies. Fatigue is no longer a signal to rest but an obstacle to override. Productivity has become a proxy for worth. In this context, the ancient Taoist principle of *wu wei*—often translated as "non-doing" or "effortless action"—does not merely appear quaint. It seems subversive. Yet it is precisely this philosophy that offers one of the most sophisticated responses to the burnout epidemic of our age.

Taoism, unlike most modern wellness ideologies, is not concerned with self-improvement. It offers no ten-step plans, no achievements to unlock. At its heart lies an invitation to *remember* what has been forgotten: that health and vitality are not manufactured through striving, but cultivated through alignment. To live in accordance with the Tao—the Way—is not to force life into submission, but to meet its current with less resistance and more attunement. *Wu wei*, then, is not passivity. It is skillful presence. It is the capacity to act without struggle, to yield without collapse, to be in motion without compulsive effort.

This philosophy begins with a radical reframing of energy itself. In the West, energy is often treated mechanistically—as fuel to be burned, as a commodity to be managed, replenished, or hacked. But Taoist traditions regard energy (or *qi*) not as a limited resource to be hoarded, but as a dynamic flow shaped by relationship: with breath, with time, with space, with season. Overexertion is not just a symptom of stress—it is a sign that one is moving *against* the Tao, out of rhythm with life's deeper harmonies.

Real-world application of *wu wei* does not require retreat to a monastery. It begins in the micro-adjustments of everyday living. Consider the case of Mei, a Shanghai-based executive who had been experiencing persistent digestive pain and insomnia. Conventional treatments yielded only marginal relief. But a Taoist medicine practitioner observed that her entire nervous system was "on the offensive"—overplanned, overstimulated, overstrategised. She was taught not just breathing techniques or acupressure, but a new approach to decision-making: to pause before acting, to move from felt-sense rather than mental compulsion. Within two months of practicing this calibrated non-doing, her pain significantly reduced. But more importantly, she reported that her internal environment had softened. She no longer mistook momentum for direction.

Taoism's most elegant expressions of *wu wei* are found in nature metaphors—water that carves stone not by force, but by constancy; bamboo that survives storms by bending, not resisting. These are not poetic flourishes. They are *functional blueprints* for resilience. In the Tao Te Ching, Laozi writes: "The soft overcomes the hard. The gentle overcomes the rigid." The nervous system, long brutalised by the myth of grind culture, responds not to pressure, but to rhythm. Taoist-informed movement practices like Qi Gong embody this insight precisely. Each movement is deliberate yet relaxed, structured yet fluid. The aim is not to train the body into submission, but to return it to coherence.

Contrast this with the dominant fitness paradigms of the West, which often treat exercise as punishment for stillness or indulgence. Taoist movement systems are not about calorie burn or muscle definition. They are about cultivating internal spaciousness. Practitioners report that after just ten minutes of slow circular arm motions, their minds quieten, their breath deepens, and a subtle joy returns—not from excitement, but from *relief*. This is what happens when action flows from being rather than anxiety.

The philosophical implications of *wu wei* extend beyond personal wellness. They challenge the very frameworks we use to approach social change, leadership, and creativity. In contrast to top-down control models, *wu wei* suggests that *effectiveness arises from congruence, not command.* A Taoist-informed therapist, for example, may say less, but listen more attentively—guiding the session not by agenda, but by attunement. Similarly, a leader practising *wu wei* learns to intervene only when necessary, trusting the intelligence of the system rather than micro-managing its every move. Paradoxically, such "inaction" often produces better outcomes than aggressive steering.

Critics argue that *wu wei* risks becoming an excuse for inaction or complacency, especially in the face of urgent crises. But this critique misunderstands the concept entirely. *Wu wei* is not indifference; it is precision. It means doing the right thing at the right time, with the right amount of effort—and only that. It is the opposite of learned helplessness. It is *disciplined receptivity.* When practiced with discernment, it fosters sharper instincts, greater efficiency, and an intuitive clarity that no to-do list can replicate.

This clarity becomes especially relevant in the realm of mental health. Many modern forms of anxiety are not rooted in trauma per se, but in overreach—a chronic misalignment between what we feel and what we force. One psychotherapist, working with clients recovering from corporate burnout, integrates Taoist principles by asking them not what they want to achieve, but *what they can allow.* In the silence that follows, clients often confront their most honest realisations—not as goals, but as invitations. This subtle pivot shifts them from coping to *re-orienting.* They begin to sense when to speak and when to stay silent, when to move and when to rest—not as binary choices, but as fluid responses shaped by context.

Even in creative fields, *wu wei* offers a rare antidote to the tyranny of hustle. Writers, musicians, and designers often report that their most inspired work emerges not when they "push through," but when they *stop interfering.* Taoist philosopher Zhuangzi described this as "fasting of the mind"—a state in which the intellect no longer dominates, and a deeper intelligence is permitted to lead. Artists trained in Taoist aesthetics are often taught to paint not what they see, but what they feel *before thought.* The brush becomes an extension of presence, not performance.

In clinical settings, especially those integrating Eastern modalities, *wu wei* is beginning to inform protocols for stress, chronic fatigue, and nervous system dysregulation. A recent study at a Shanghai integrative medicine centre explored how non-linear interventions—such as mindful waiting, breath-led movement, and non-outcome-based therapy—produced statistically significant reductions in anxiety and cortisol levels. The insight here is less about the specific modality and more about the *orientation to action.* By doing less, patients could feel more. And by feeling more, they could heal with less internal resistance.

Yet perhaps the most radical element of *wu wei* is what it demands of the practitioner: *trust.* Trust that life has its own intelligence. Trust that rest is not regression. Trust that outcomes need not be chased, only met with readiness. This is profoundly difficult in a culture trained to equate stillness with failure. But Taoist practice begins where control ends. It is not about learning to dominate complexity, but learning to dance with it.

In the current climate—ecological, political, psychological—this principle holds particular urgency. Our systems are overheated, our leaders overcorrecting, our bodies overstimulated. Taoism does not propose a utopia. It offers something quieter and perhaps more sustainable: a way of being that does not require collapse before change. *Wu wei* is not the abandonment of responsibility; it is the maturation of response.

To adopt the Tao of doing less is not to withdraw from life, but to move through it differently. It is to let actions be shaped not by fear or compulsion, but by resonance. It is to understand that sometimes, the most transformative act is not an intervention, but an interruption—a space where the world, and our place within it, can recalibrate without force.

In this sense, *wu wei* is not just philosophy. It is medicine. And its dosage is absence: of urgency, of overreach, of noise. What remains is not emptiness, but clarity. And from clarity, vitality.

Movement That Listens

Most modern fitness regimes are predicated on command: push harder, burn more, go faster. Bodies are sculpted as if they are objects of control, tools of performance, or liabilities to correct. Yet when movement begins from listening rather than imposition, something ancient stirs—a form of intelligence that predates exercise as we know it. This is not about calories or cardiovascular output. It is about dialogue. In traditions like Qi Gong, tai chi, and other mindful movement practices, the body is not pushed but invited. *These are not disciplines of domination—they are practices of devotion.*

To move in this way is to dismantle the hierarchy between mind and body. In Western paradigms, the mind instructs, the body obeys. In Qi Gong, the reverse often occurs: the body speaks first, and the mind follows. This inversion is not aesthetic; it is functional. Where conventional movement pushes through sensation, mindful movement *pauses* within it. Tension becomes a signal, not a nuisance. Fatigue is acknowledged, not overridden. Each gesture becomes a gesture of listening.

Qi Gong—translated roughly as "energy cultivation"—is often dismissed in mainstream wellness culture as slow or ornamental. But within its deliberate tempo lies an extraordinary potency. The slow, rhythmic coordination of breath, posture, and intention is not merely therapeutic—it is diagnostic. Practitioners learn to detect stagnation not through symptoms, but through felt-sense: where breath skips, where joints resist, where energy dissipates. One senior practitioner, trained in the Beijing lineage, describes Qi Gong as "a means of reacquainting the body with its own subtle grammar." He tells the story of a corporate client who came seeking stress relief. After months of practice, her migraines had reduced—but more importantly, her relationship to time had changed. "She stopped hurrying," he said. "Not just physically, but psychologically."

The practice of tai chi similarly defies the modern assumption that health must be effortful. Originally developed as a martial art, tai chi has evolved into a profoundly restorative movement form that marries opposites: strength with softness, intention with receptivity. Movements that appear gentle carry a precise internal architecture; what looks relaxed is, in fact, rigorously attentive. The practitioner is never idle but never straining. This equilibrium—between alertness and ease—is what renders tai chi uniquely potent for nervous system regulation. Studies have shown its efficacy in reducing hypertension, improving balance, and modulating cortisol levels. But the deeper impact is not easily measurable. Tai chi reorganises the psyche by re-patterning the body's engagement with gravity, breath, and space.

The real significance of these practices, however, lies not just in what they do to the body, but in how they reconfigure our orientation to embodiment itself. When movement becomes a *form of presence* rather than production, the entire notion of wellness shifts. Exercise ceases to be a means of self-optimisation. It becomes a way of remembering: that vitality is not something we extract from the body, but something we co-create with it.

Western physiotherapy and somatic psychology are increasingly recognising this. Thomas Hanna, who coined the term "somatics," argued that modern disconnection from the body is not anatomical, but perceptual. We stop *feeling* ourselves. Qi Gong and tai chi offer a direct antidote—not by demanding more, but by demanding *less*. They train perception, not exertion. And in doing so, they awaken a kind of kinaesthetic empathy: with oneself, and with the environment. Movements are tuned to the rhythms of wind, season, breath. The boundary between organism and world softens. *The body no longer performs; it participates.*

This participatory ethic is central to the deeper philosophy that informs mindful movement: that health is not a private achievement, but a relational state. Just as Qi Gong seeks to harmonise the body's meridians, it also seeks to attune the practitioner to larger flows—ecological, social, temporal. One practitioner described her morning routine not as "a workout" but as "listening to the weather through my joints." Such phrasing may seem esoteric to the uninitiated, but its implications are deeply grounded. In cultures where such movement traditions persist, illness is not treated solely as biochemical failure but as a sign of dissonance—between person and pattern, body and world.

There is also a political subtext here. To reclaim slowness, softness, and non-linear motion in a culture obsessed with speed, efficiency, and symmetry is itself a radical act. Mindful movement resists not only the mechanisation of the body, but the commodification of health. It offers instead a practice rooted in agency and attention. Practitioners are not patients nor clients, but participants in their own unfolding. There is no guru dictating from above. The teacher, if present, models *how* to feel, not *what* to do.

This is not to romanticise these traditions or strip them of rigour. Both Qi Gong and tai chi require consistency, discipline, and an ongoing relationship with subtlety. But unlike conventional exercise, where more is often better, mindful movement introduces the ethic of *enough*. A session might end not when one is exhausted, but when coherence is restored. This redefinition of thresholds is especially relevant for individuals navigating chronic fatigue, trauma, or neurodivergence—populations for whom standard movement prescriptions often do more harm than good. Mindful movement creates space for nuance, for pacing, for dignity.

Importantly, these traditions also challenge the neurocentric model of embodiment. Where Western biomedicine often locates consciousness in the brain, Qi Gong and tai chi treat awareness as dispersed—located in breath, blood, fascia. The practitioner is taught to feel from the centre of the palm, the base of the spine, the soles of the feet. One teacher of the Five Animal Frolics—a classical Qi Gong set—tells students to "breathe through your kidneys." While not anatomically literal, the instruction fosters an embodied imagination that reconnects physiology to feeling. *This is not mysticism; it is pedagogy.* It cultivates sensory literacy in a culture that has been largely numbed.

Emerging neuroscience supports these insights. Polyvagal theory, for instance, posits that the vagus nerve—the main conduit of parasympathetic tone—is highly responsive to slow, rhythmic movement. Practices like Qi Gong and tai chi, which integrate exhalation with spiral motion and open-focus attention, directly engage this system. The result is not simply relaxation, but *co-regulation*: a state in which the body feels safe enough to repair, rewire, and relate.

What distinguishes these forms from casual stretching or mindfulness apps is their *cosmology*. Movement is not isolated from ethics or worldview. Each gesture embodies a principle: rooting before rising, yielding before initiating, conserving before releasing. These are not just physical cues. They are philosophical commitments, trained into tissue. Practised daily, they reshape one's metabolism of life itself. Conflict, urgency, ambition—each is met with different muscle tone, different breath pattern, different postural bias. Over time, the practitioner ceases to compartmentalise their movement from their living. They do not move to escape life; they move to *become more porous to it.*

The phrase "movement that listens" is thus not poetic hyperbole. It is an instruction. It asks: what if every motion were a response, not an assertion? What if wellness began not with intervention, but with intimacy? In these quiet forms of devotion, the body is neither enemy nor idol—it is companion. And in moving with it, rather than on top of it, we recover something more essential than fitness: *relationship.*

This is what Qi Gong and tai chi offer—not choreography, but conversation. Not optimisation, but orientation. And for a world that has mistaken noise for vitality, this listening might be the most urgent movement of all.

Chapter 7
The Mind as Garden: Reweaving Cognitive and Emotional Ecology

Mental health is seldom confined to the workings of the mind alone. It is, rather, an ecology—woven from cognitive, emotional, relational, and even ancestral threads. The metaphors we have inherited for the psyche tend towards the linear and mechanical: the mind as machine, to be repaired; as software, to be reprogrammed. Such images, though neat, fall short of capturing the organic, tangled reality of lived experience. Thought, like earth, is altered by weather. Emotional habits are not purely personal—they carry the imprint of cultural inheritance, passed down like language or a family mannerism. This chapter offers another frame: to regard the psyche not as a static object but as a living ecosystem. Some thoughts are not our own. Some moods belong to another time. Some wounds will not yield to willpower alone.

To tend the mind as one might tend a garden is no quaint indulgence—it is an act of skill and discipline. It asks for observation, curiosity, and the recognition that what shows itself—anxiety, the inner voice of derision, the steady hum of self-doubt—often springs from seeds sown in soil we did not choose. What may look like a failing in character can, on closer inspection, reveal itself as an inherited survival strategy. A habit of hyper-vigilance may be the distant echo of war, migration, or family instability. The conviction that one must earn love through output may not be an idiosyncrasy of personality at all, but rather a reflection of a culture addicted to productivity as proof of worth. The work, then, is not to turn the self into a diagnostic specimen, but to see it within its rightful context.

Modern studies in epigenetics and intergenerational trauma now affirm what many older healing traditions have held for centuries: that our patterns are passed along not only through stories, but in the body's own chemistry. Neuroscience shows how beliefs shape the structure of the brain; somatic therapy reveals that unresolved emotional history resides not just in thought, but in flesh. The mind–

body divide—once a cornerstone of Western psychiatry—is rapidly crumbling. Still, mainstream mental health treatment often clings to cognitive-behavioural approaches: locate the thought, challenge it, replace it. These methods have their worth, yet they skim the surface. They rarely reach into the deeper ecological networks from which thoughts grow. True healing is not merely a matter of rewiring; it is an act of reweaving.

Four themes will guide this chapter's reorientation of mental resilience. First: not every thought is truly yours. Cultural conditioning, family stories, systemic bias, and the residue of generational strain form the backdrop of cognition. What feels like a personal failing may instead be a symptom of a shared inheritance. Recognising this does not absolve responsibility—it sharpens it, offering clarity over what is ours to work with and what can, with care, be laid back in the hands of history. Consider the woman raised in a lineage where emotion was stifled; she may find tears tangled with shame. Therapy alone may falter here unless the cultural and familial threads are drawn into view. Healing, in such cases, becomes less about repair and more about excavation.

Second: the inner critic, so often cast as the villain, is frequently a bodily stress reflex in disguise. Persistent self-attack can be the internalised hand of control, forged when external safety was scarce. The refrain of "you are not enough" is often the ghost of a time when love was conditional, security fragile, or achievement a necessity for survival. Rather than silencing the critic, we can trace its voice back to its origin. Somatic compassion—placing a hand over the heart, naming the bodily sensation behind the words, speaking to the critic as one would to a frightened child—begins to quiet its urgency. This part of the self is not an enemy, but an old sentinel who has never stopped bracing for impact.

Third: narrative as a form of medicine. Just as trauma fractures the coherence of identity, the telling of one's story—when done well—can help to reassemble it. Yet not every story heals. The dominant narratives we inherit about strength, success, gender, or emotion are often reductive, even colonising. Practices drawn from indigenous storytelling and depth psychology invite a re-authoring of experience into more spacious and truthful forms. Writing, speaking aloud, or engaging in therapeutic dialogue are not mere acts of expression—they are processes by which psychic waste can be turned into fertile ground for understanding. A survivor of emotional abuse, for example, might one day reframe her past, not as a chronicle of damage, but as a testament to boundary-setting and ancestral endurance. This is not the invention of a new truth, but the unveiling of a deeper one that had been obscured.

Finally, the stance of sufficiency. In a culture steeped in capitalism and constant comparison, the mind is awash with scarcity. "I haven't done enough. I'm not there yet. I don't have enough." This quiet starvation drains vitality, masquerading as ambition. Research from positive psychology, Buddhist thought, and neuroplasticity converge on the understanding that gratitude, contentment, and rest are not luxuries but skills—ones that can be trained. Simple practices, like ending the day by noting not achievements but completions—what was lived, what was felt, what was met—can, over time, soften the reflex to grasp. Slowly, the nervous system learns that it is safe to stop running.

Together, these four perspectives offer a frame rather than a formula. They allow us to move away from pathologising the inner landscape and towards caring for it. The garden metaphor is deliberate. Gardens do require tending, but they also need space. Some growth must be wild; some healing happens where we cannot see it. To acknowledge this is not to lapse into sentimentalism or avoid reality—it is to accept that the psyche flourishes not through relentless correction, but through cycles of nourishment and rest.

By the close of this chapter, the reader will carry away both conceptual and practical tools: somatic practices to soothe the inner critic, journaling prompts to reframe inherited stories, embodied rituals to cultivate sufficiency, and insights to untangle personal identity from inherited thought. More than that, they will hold a reimagined definition of mental wellness—not as a permanent state of calm or cheer, but as a capacity to engage well with the ecosystem within.

This is not an instruction to fix the mind. It is an invitation to rewild it—to break down what no longer serves, to water what longs to grow. And to remember that the most intelligent aspect of your psyche may not be your thoughts at all, but your ability to witness, tend, and transform them. You are not only a thinker; you are a cultivator. The rest is practice.

Not All Thoughts Are Yours

Most people live their entire lives assuming their thoughts belong to them. This belief—that what we think originates solely from within—forms the foundation of modern psychology and self-help culture alike. It is the logic behind countless affirmations, cognitive-behavioural interventions, and well-meaning advice urging us to "change our mindset" or "reframe the story." But what if some of those thoughts didn't begin with you? What if the voice in your head isn't simply *yours*, but an echo—an inherited pattern of vigilance, shame, or perfectionism passed down through generations or absorbed unconsciously from culture? When we take our thoughts at face value, we risk treating inherited wounds as personal flaws. We pathologise our response without investigating its source. *Not all thoughts are yours* is not a metaphor—it is a rigorous starting point for healing.

Contemporary neuroscience and trauma research have begun to validate what traditional systems of wisdom have long known: thoughts, like behaviours and emotional patterns, can be inherited. Epigenetics has shown us that stress responses—particularly those resulting from trauma, poverty, and displacement—can be encoded in gene expression and transmitted across generations. What a grandparent lived through during war or migration might shape the stress thresholds and default reactions of their descendants. This is not mere sentimentality; it is biological fact. When a person carries chronic anxiety despite a relatively stable life, the explanation may not lie in their biography, but in their lineage. One study from the Max Planck Institute, for example, found that descendants of Holocaust survivors exhibited measurable changes in stress hormone regulation. These changes affected their emotional regulation and cortisol response, even though they had not lived through the trauma themselves. *Your nervous system remembers what your mind has never known.*

And beyond the intergenerational lies the cultural. Thought habits often mirror the assumptions and survival mechanisms of the societies we live in. A hyper-capitalist society will promote internal scripts of productivity, self-judgement, and comparison. In such a context, a person who slows down, questions their ambition, or feels fulfilled without achievement might experience guilt—not because something is wrong with them, but because they are deviating from the implicit rules of their environment. The thought "I'm not doing enough" may not be evidence of laziness or fear of success, but a symptom of a cultural trance. From a therapeutic standpoint, this insight matters profoundly. If we misdiagnose cultural indoctrination as personal pathology, we end up treating the individual while leaving the system untouched. *Healing, in this light, becomes an act of cultural inquiry—not just personal change.*

To illustrate, consider Maya, a high-performing medical student who began experiencing debilitating perfectionism and self-doubt. Her therapy focused initially on cognitive restructuring, attempting to replace her inner critic with positive affirmations. But nothing shifted. It wasn't until she explored her family history that deeper patterns emerged: her grandmother had survived Partition, her mother had raised children while navigating racism in academia, and both had linked worth with impeccable performance. Maya wasn't merely overthinking; she was embodying a generational demand to succeed in order to survive. Her inner critic was not irrational—it was historical. Recognising this didn't erase the thought, but it transformed her relationship to it. *She stopped trying to silence the voice and began listening to its origins.*

What we commonly call "limiting beliefs" are often adaptive beliefs—crafted in contexts that made them necessary. For instance, the belief "I can't trust anyone" may be maladaptive in a safe relationship, but it likely served a protective function in a home where betrayal or instability were the norm. Unlearning such thoughts requires more than mental override; it requires *relational repair.* And here lies the danger of modern affirmation culture: it attempts to overwrite before it understands. The deeper question is not "Is this thought true?" but *"Who taught me this, and what were they surviving?"* This shift reframes healing as inquiry, not intervention.

This is where trauma-informed mindfulness, somatic therapy, and depth-oriented psychologies intersect. These modalities teach that to disidentify from inherited thoughts, we must bring the body into the process. Thought patterns often have somatic anchors: the tightening in the chest that arrives with guilt, the clench in the jaw accompanying self-judgement, the shallow breath tied to urgency. Unlearning requires noticing. Noticing requires *slowing down.* By mapping where certain thoughts live in the body, we begin to dislodge them not only cognitively, but physiologically. This is not about becoming thoughtless; it is about creating enough spaciousness to discern which thoughts are *helpful*, which are *ancestral*, and which are *indoctrinated.*

There is also a collective and ethical dimension here. In multicultural societies shaped by histories of colonialism, caste, racism, and patriarchy, many thought habits are actually survival adaptations to systemic oppression. The thought "I must work twice as hard to be respected" is not baseless anxiety for many Black professionals—it is lived reality. Similarly, the internalised belief among many women that being assertive makes them "difficult" is a product of centuries of social conditioning, not a flaw in character. The implication for mental health care is urgent: we must be cautious not to label adaptive responses as irrational simply because they are no longer convenient. *Context determines function.* What may seem like a cognitive distortion could, under the lens of lived experience, be revealed as a protective truth.

So how do we begin the work of discernment? Not through quick fixes, but through practices of deep listening and slow unlearning. Journaling becomes a powerful tool, not for recounting events, but for investigating thought lineage. Asking "Whose voice is this?" or "What fear is this thought protecting me from?" allows us to name inherited patterns. Somatic tracking—pausing to feel what happens in the body when a thought arises—grounds the inquiry. And group work or therapy spaces that centre cultural and ancestral awareness can offer the validation needed to release shame. There is a unique power in discovering that what you carry is not *yours alone*, and therefore, not yours to hold forever.

Reclaiming authorship over thought doesn't mean having perfect control. It means having intimate familiarity with the forces that shape your inner landscape. It means learning the difference between a thought that emerges from presence and one that echoes a script written decades or centuries ago. It means learning to say, "That is not mine," with clarity and without blame. And it means cultivating the humility to know that sometimes, the most harmful beliefs persist not because they are true, but because they went unexamined for too long.

Ultimately, to say that not all thoughts are yours is not to diminish responsibility—it is to deepen it. When we see thought as a communal, historical, and somatic phenomenon, we can approach mental health not as a solo journey of optimisation, but as a process of reconnection. Reconnection to body. Reconnection to lineage. Reconnection to truth. And most radically, perhaps, reconnection to silence—the space between thoughts, where something wiser may be waiting.

The Inner Critic as a Stress Response

The voice of the inner critic is rarely just a voice. It is a tightening of the chest before sending an email, a flinch in the gut when receiving praise, a burning drive to prove oneself even in the absence of external pressure. It is not simply a thought that says *"You're not enough"*—it is a full-body signal that something is unsafe. Though commonly framed as a personality flaw or unhelpful habit, the inner critic is more accurately understood as a survival strategy. It arises from a nervous system trained to anticipate rejection, disappointment, or danger. *It is not a malfunction—it is an adaptation.*

This reframe is crucial because it alters how we respond to the inner critic. Rather than engaging in a cognitive duel, trying to override or silence it with affirmations, we begin to ask deeper questions: What is this voice protecting me from? When did it first appear? And how does my body respond when it speaks? These questions pivot us away from internal warfare toward compassionate inquiry. They reveal that for many people, especially those who've experienced developmental trauma, systemic marginalisation, or chronic instability, self-criticism is not self-hatred—it is self-protection rehearsed over decades.

The origins of the inner critic often lie in relational dynamics during formative years. A child exposed to unpredictable caregivers, punitive authority figures, or high expectations learns that internal vigilance is safer than external vulnerability. If perfection was rewarded and mistakes punished—explicitly or implicitly—the nervous system begins to equate self-worth with flawlessness. Over time, the internal voice that anticipates critique becomes preferable to the real thing. The logic is simple: *If I criticise myself first, others won't have to.* In this way, the inner critic develops not to destroy us, but to keep us safe within a particular relational economy. It is the body's way of staying one step ahead of shame.

Modern stress research supports this interpretation. Studies in psychoneuroimmunology show that self-critical thinking activates the same neurobiological pathways as social threat. When a person berates themselves—calling themselves lazy, stupid, or a failure—the amygdala responds as though an external predator is present. Cortisol levels rise. The body prepares for attack. This suggests that self-attack is not an internal monologue—it is a full physiological event. The body cannot distinguish between being insulted by someone else and being insulted by oneself. From a therapeutic standpoint, this insight is monumental: chronic self-criticism is not just a psychological burden, it is a somatic stressor. *It keeps the body in a loop of low-grade threat, making true rest impossible.*

To effectively address the inner critic, we must look beyond mindset interventions and toward somatic compassion. This does not mean replacing self-judgement with hollow positivity. It means cultivating a nervous system that knows how to feel safe without the need for constant vigilance. One powerful framework comes from the field of somatic experiencing, which views healing as a process of renegotiating threat responses in the body. When the critic arises, the invitation is not to argue with it but to locate its echo in the body: Where does the tension land? What posture does it evoke? What emotion lies beneath it—fear, grief, anger? This embodied awareness shifts the relationship from identification ("*I am a failure*") to observation ("*This is a familiar stress response trying to protect me*").

Practical interventions include orienting exercises—pausing to look around the room and name what is physically present—to bring the body into the here and now. Gentle touch, such as placing a hand over the heart or belly, can cue a parasympathetic response, especially when paired with phrases like *"This is hard, and I'm here."* These gestures may seem small, but they signal to the nervous system that safety is possible without self-punishment. Over time, this builds a new repertoire of responses: instead of tightening when we fall short, we soften. Instead of preparing to fight ourselves, we prepare to listen.

One case that illustrates this transformation is Lila, a corporate executive who entered therapy with complaints of burnout and self-sabotage. She described herself as "driven but miserable," waking each day with a sense of dread despite outward success. Her inner critic, she said, was "always on," criticising everything from her voice in meetings to her performance in relationships. Traditional coaching had urged her to reframe her thoughts, but nothing stuck. When her work turned somatic, something shifted. During one session, she realised that her critical voice carried the cadence of her father—whose love was conditional on achievement. Her shoulders tensed every time she recalled his disappointment. By learning to sense these micro-responses and meet them with compassion, Lila began to uncouple success from survival. The voice didn't disappear, but it lost its grip. *She was no longer entranced by its urgency.*

This story underscores a vital point: the inner critic can be a reliable indicator of where healing is needed. It often surfaces most aggressively when we are on the verge of change—when we try something unfamiliar, set a boundary, or rest without justification. It rushes in not because we are weak, but because a part of us still believes that deviation from the old rules is dangerous. Rather than seeing this as sabotage, we can see it as a call for integration. *The critic is not the enemy. It is a part of us that is still afraid.*

This perspective has powerful implications in educational and organisational settings. In high-stress environments, self-criticism is often misread as commitment or humility. People who internalise failure are praised for being self-aware, when in reality they are eroding their capacity for resilience. Leaders and educators must learn to distinguish between accountability and self-attack. The former supports growth; the latter diminishes it. Promoting cultures of psychological safety—not just through policies, but through relational practices—is essential. Compassionate feedback, permission to make mistakes, and models of self-kindness are not soft practices—they are neurological necessities for long-term performance.

There is also a sociopolitical dimension worth noting. The prevalence of the inner critic is not randomly distributed. Research shows that women, people of colour, and LGBTQ+ individuals are more likely to struggle with chronic self-criticism, particularly in professional or academic settings. This is not because of individual pathology, but because of systemic gaslighting—years of being implicitly or explicitly told that their presence must be justified. For these populations, the inner critic often doubles as an internalised voice of marginalisation. Healing, therefore, must include not just self-compassion, but *structural validation.* It is not enough to be kind to oneself in private—we must also challenge the environments that provoke self-attack in the first place.

So where does this leave us? Not with a neatly resolved mindset, but with an invitation to relate to ourselves differently. The question is not *"How do I stop criticising myself?"* but *"Can I hold the part of me that learned to criticise with compassion?"* This is the paradox of healing: we cannot bully the bully into silence. But we can meet it with enough patience, truth, and somatic safety that it begins to trust a new way of being. That it begins to loosen. That it learns, over time, that vigilance is no longer required.

The inner critic, then, is not a flaw to be fixed, but a doorway. A signal. A remnant of love distorted by fear. And when we approach it with the respect and nuance it deserves, it can become something else entirely: a teacher. A reminder of where we've been. And a companion on the way to where we're going—if we dare to lead with something softer.

Story as Medicine

What we believe about ourselves is rarely based on fact. It is based on the stories we have repeated—aloud, in memory, in silence—so often that they begin to feel like identity. I am the one who always ruins things. I can't handle conflict. I'm too much. These phrases are not truths; they are internalised narratives, shaped by culture, context, and trauma. And while they may begin as coping strategies, over time they become scripts that limit our capacity to heal. *To change how we feel, we must change how we narrate.*

This is the premise of narrative therapy, a psychotherapeutic approach that treats language not as a reflection of reality but as a force that constructs it. Developed in the 1980s by Michael White and David Epston, narrative therapy centres on the idea that people are not their problems—they are the authors of meaning. Problems are external, stories are mutable, and healing lies not in suppressing painful experiences but in reauthoring the plotlines that frame them. It is not the trauma that breaks us, but the interpretation that calcifies in its wake.

In the clinical context, narrative therapy involves deconstructing "problem-saturated" narratives and amplifying "preferred stories"—alternative accounts that highlight resilience, values, or moments of agency. For instance, a client who frames themselves as inherently broken might, through dialogue, rediscover a time they acted with strength or compassion, even amidst suffering. This moment becomes a narrative thread worth following. Not to deny the pain, but to *relocate the self* within a richer, more multidimensional frame.

The power of this work lies in its relationality. In traditional Western psychology, the self is often treated as an isolated entity. Narrative therapy disrupts that assumption, treating identity as relational, cultural, and temporal. It recognises that the stories we carry are not always ours by choice. They are inherited—passed down from parents, reinforced by schooling, magnified by media. When someone says, "I'm not good enough," that voice often echoes a family lineage of scarcity or a societal norm of perfectionism. To heal, we must *decolonise our narratives*—tease apart what was chosen from what was imposed.

One of the most accessible and powerful ways to begin this work outside of therapy is through reflective writing. Journaling, when approached not as a diary of events but as an act of authorship, can be a tool for narrative reconfiguration. The simple act of writing a moment from the past in the third person—"she was terrified, but she stood her ground"—can begin to rewire identification. It creates space between the experience and the self. That space is where transformation begins. This is not performative gratitude or positive thinking. It is *grief-informed revision.* It is learning to look again, and to look with care.

Consider the practice of mythic retelling, a form of narrative alchemy rooted in archetypal psychology. This approach invites individuals to rewrite their experiences as if they were myths—placing themselves in the role of protagonist, naming obstacles as dragons or deserts, and asking what the story demands for resolution. This isn't childish fantasy; it is *a reactivation of the imagination as a healing faculty.* Carl Jung called myth the "collective dream of a culture." When we locate our individual struggles within universal patterns—exile, return, rebirth—we stop pathologising ourselves and begin to feel part of something larger.

This is particularly powerful in contexts where trauma has fractured continuity. Survivors of abuse, war, systemic oppression or migration often describe feeling "outside of time"—disconnected from a coherent narrative of who they are. Story work can re-establish temporal integrity, bridging the past, present and future. It allows one to say: *That happened, it shaped me, but it does not define me. I am more than one chapter.*

A vivid example comes from a narrative therapist working with recently resettled refugees in Europe. One participant, a former teacher who had lost everything, described himself only in the language of failure. Through facilitated storytelling, he began to reconnect with his past not only as a sequence of losses, but as a tapestry of roles—father, educator, survivor. Eventually, he wrote a short story in which his experience was reframed as a journey of integrity and courage, with a protagonist who refused to abandon kindness despite cruelty. That story became a reference point he could return to—a stabilising myth that honoured both pain and agency. *This is the medicine of story: it provides continuity where life has been broken.*

But not all story work is therapeutic in the clinical sense. In indigenous and traditional healing systems, stories are used as vehicles of teaching and transformation. They are not merely reflections of experience—they *shape experience.* In many African, Native American, and First Nations communities, healing stories are told not to explain but to embody wisdom. Their power lies not in factuality but in transmission. They move through the nervous system in ways logic cannot. To listen to a story told in ceremony is to participate in a ritual of collective meaning-making. The story becomes a container for pain, insight, and cultural memory.

Modern therapeutic culture often neglects this communal dimension. Yet the epidemic of isolation that underpins much chronic stress cannot be resolved through private insight alone. We need communal storytelling practices—not just in therapy rooms, but in schools, organisations, families. Story circles, when facilitated with skill and consent, can be spaces where people re-encounter themselves in the eyes of others. They reveal that the most private shame often carries universal notes. As one facilitator said, "When someone else names your story, you realise it never belonged to you alone."

This raises an ethical dimension: storytelling is powerful medicine, but it must be used responsibly. Not every trauma must be narrated to be healed. There is a risk in commodifying story—turning it into content, performance, or currency in a culture that rewards vulnerability on display. True narrative healing respects boundaries. It centres *agency*, not disclosure. It asks not just what happened, but whether telling it serves the teller. In this way, storytelling becomes less about confession and more about *integration.* It is not about impressing an audience—it is about restoring coherence within.

A related pitfall is the temptation to impose linearity. People often feel pressure to wrap their stories in tidy resolutions—to show growth, transformation, redemption. But healing is rarely linear. Sometimes the most honest story is unfinished. Sometimes we need to speak from the middle, from the confusion, from the ache that hasn't found meaning yet. Holding space for *unfinished stories*—without rushing to interpret or solve—is one of the most generous things we can do for ourselves and others.

For those seeking to begin this work, a simple practice is the use of dual journaling: two columns on a page, one for "dominant story" and one for "preferred story." On the left, write what the inner critic or inherited narrative says—*"I always fail at relationships."* On the right, write a moment that disrupts that script—*"I stayed through a friend's grief even when it was hard."* This practice doesn't aim to replace one with the other, but to introduce complexity. *Healing lies in multiplicity, not reduction.*

Ultimately, story as medicine is not about crafting a perfect narrative. It is about reclaiming authorship over the meanings that shape our lives. It is about recognising that even amidst the stories we've inherited—of scarcity, trauma, inadequacy—we have the right to write something new. And perhaps more importantly, we have the right to leave certain stories behind. Not because they are untrue, but because they are too small to hold who we are becoming.

The Mindset of Enough

Scarcity is rarely about resources. It is about perception. A person with three months of savings can feel safer than someone with six figures in the bank, and a child with one toy may feel more joy than an adult with a garage full of gadgets. The mindset of scarcity—*there is not enough, I am not enough, it won't be enough*—is not an economic condition. It is a psychological imprint, often inherited and unconsciously reinforced. It is also one of the most potent contributors to chronic stress in the modern world.

The scarcity mindset is not merely a pessimistic outlook; it is a nervous system state. When one perceives a constant deficit—of time, attention, love, money, worth—the body enters subtle survival mode. The sympathetic nervous system stays activated, digestion slows, creative thinking narrows, and relational safety erodes. The result is a perpetual low-grade anxiety that masquerades as ambition or realism. People living with this mindset often overwork, overthink, overconsume, or overextend, not because they are driven, but because they are afraid—afraid that stopping means slipping behind, being forgotten, or losing control. *Scarcity doesn't push us toward excellence—it pulls us away from presence.*

Contrast this with sufficiency: a state of internal orientation that says, *I have what I need for this moment. I can meet life from a place of stability rather than scramble.* Sufficiency is not complacency. It is not a denial of challenges or the pursuit of growth. Rather, it is the recognition that security, belonging, and value begin *inside*, and that no external acquisition can replace a grounded sense of enoughness. This shift from scarcity to sufficiency is not merely philosophical—it is *physiological.* When one internalises sufficiency, the nervous system downregulates, cortisol decreases, the vagus nerve activates, and the body re-enters relational and creative flow.

One of the central insights from somatic psychology is that perception precedes cognition. You can read every affirmation about abundance, but if your body is still wired for famine—emotional, material, or existential—you will not feel safe. This is why cultivating the mindset of enough requires more than cognitive reframing. It requires *embodied practice.* It asks us to literally *teach the body* that the emergency has passed.

A simple yet profound exercise begins with breath and interoception. Sit still, close your eyes, and feel into the internal landscape. Ask quietly: *What am I craving right now? What do I fear I do not have?* Let the answers emerge without judgement. Then, ask a second question: *What evidence exists in this moment that I am resourced?* Perhaps it is a warm room, a quiet space, a heartbeat, a breath, a friend nearby. As you name each resource, place your hand on your chest or abdomen and anchor the awareness. Over time, this practice builds what trauma therapist Resmaa Menakem calls *a settled body*—one that can perceive sufficiency without being overridden by ancestral alarm.

It is worth pausing here to consider how often scarcity is not personal but cultural. Modern capitalism runs on the engine of insufficiency. It must, in order to sell. If every person felt whole, centred, and worthy, the demand for self-optimisation products, status goods, or fear-driven news would collapse. Scarcity is curated—through advertising, through metrics of comparison, through productivity myths. A teenager today may scroll through 500 idealised images before breakfast, each whispering: *You are falling behind.* Against this backdrop, the choice to practise enoughness is not self-help. *It is rebellion.*

In contemplative traditions—Buddhism, Taoism, Yogic philosophy—sufficiency is a central pillar of wellbeing. In Yogic ethics, the principle of *Santosha* (contentment) invites one to rest in the adequacy of the present, while still acknowledging aspiration. In Taoism, non-striving (*wu wei*) emerges from recognising that life unfolds best when not forcefully grasped. In Buddhist practice, the relinquishment of grasping is seen not as loss but as liberation. Across these systems, *enoughness is not resignation. It is return.*

In clinical practice, the scarcity mindset often surfaces in the language clients use: "I'm running out of time." "I'll never be where I need to be." "It's too late for me." These are not facts—they are cognitive residues of chronic dysregulation. In therapeutic settings, simply slowing down the pace of speech, or inviting a pause between sentences, can begin to recalibrate urgency. One clinician recounts a moment where a client, always speaking rapidly, was invited to take three breaths before responding. In the silence, tears came—not from sadness, but from the shock of encountering spaciousness. The insight that followed: *I didn't know there was room for me to exist without performing.* That moment marked the beginning of healing—not because her external conditions changed, but because her inner architecture did.

To actively shift into a sufficiency mindset, structured reflection can be helpful. One exercise, adapted from Joanna Macy's "Work That Reconnects," asks participants to list not what they lack, but what supports them. Categories include people, practices, places, memories, and inner qualities. Writing these out can begin to disrupt the default orientation of deficit. Another practice involves identifying the thresholds of "enough"—What is enough rest? Enough income? Enough social connection?—and tracking how often those thresholds are internally overridden by stories of comparison or scarcity.

Yet, one of the most under-recognised forms of scarcity is not about money or time—it is *relational enoughness*. Many people operate from a deep fear of being too much or not enough in their relationships. They apologise for emotions, suppress needs, or perform roles to remain acceptable. This relational scarcity creates chronic stress—not only because it exhausts the nervous system, but because it denies the body the core regulation of secure attachment. Cultivating relational sufficiency begins with the radical belief that *your presence is not a burden*. Practising self-disclosure, setting boundaries, or simply being witnessed without fixing are all ways of restoring relational abundance. Not because others change, but because you stop translating needs as flaws.

Importantly, the mindset of enough is not a static destination. It is a daily discipline, a practice of returning. Like breath, it must be renewed. It is not a matter of never feeling lack, but of noticing when you slip into contraction, and gently widening back out. This is where mindfulness becomes essential—not as a trendy technique, but as a mechanism of *inner attunement*. When you catch the thought, "I should be further along," you can ask, "Who told me that?" and then decide whether the story is worth keeping.

Sufficiency also requires collective imagination. It asks: What would systems look like if they were built on the assumption that people are enough? How would workplaces change if rest was seen as productive? How would education shift if we nurtured capacity rather than performance? What would public policy look like if human dignity wasn't contingent on output? These questions are not abstract. They are blueprints for cultural repair.

Scarcity is not just exhausting—it is corrosive. It erodes trust, breeds competition, and fractures our sense of belonging. The mindset of enough, by contrast, is generative. It makes space for collaboration, creativity, and care. It allows us to celebrate others without self-erasure. It teaches us to savour without hoarding, to strive without panic, and to rest without guilt.

We live in a world engineered for speed, comparison, and craving. To cultivate sufficiency within that world is not naive—it is necessary. Because until we learn to say, with clarity and conviction, *this is enough*, we will remain hostage to the illusion that we are never quite whole. And nothing—not success, not status, not self-improvement—can heal a nervous system that has forgotten what it feels like to arrive.

Chapter 8
Sacred Slowness: Rituals to Reclaim Time and Rhythm

Slowness is neither a failure of discipline nor a dalliance for the idle. It is a potent remedy—one that our urgency-drunk civilisation has largely forgotten. We live in a culture where speed is lionised and stillness regarded with suspicion, yet the deepest forms of repair—grieving, healing, loving, digesting life itself—unfold only in the spaciousness that modern capitalism cannot quantify. To reclaim time is, in a sense, to reclaim one's very self. This is not simply a matter of optimising calendars, but of reimagining what time is and how it wishes to move through us.

For most, time today is linear, scarce, and transactional. It is diced into grids, measured against productivity targets, and swallowed whole by obligations. Such time is not benign—it is extracted, designed to pull the body away from its own rhythms, to sever rest from the psyche, and to banish the sacred from the everyday. The metaphors betray the mindset: we "spend" time, "waste" time, "invest" time—as though its only value lay in economic return. But before time was treated as currency, it was ceremony. It was the sun and the moon, the pulse of the tides, the cadence of planting and harvest, woven into songlines and rites. Across Indigenous, Vedic, Taoist, and countless other traditions, time was not managed but honoured. To live well with time was to live well with the world.

So, what might it mean to restore such a relationship—not abstractly, but in the folds of daily life? Sacred slowness is not merely doing less; it is doing with full presence. It asks us to look for the sacred not in rare, curated experiences but in the humble, steady rituals that hold our days together: smoothing oil into the skin at dawn, lighting a candle at nightfall, letting tea steep without hurrying, scribbling thoughts before sleep. These small, repeated gestures become anchors in the flow of hours, signalling to the nervous system: you are not merely enduring today—you are inhabiting it.

Ritual, here, is not psychological ornamentation but biological necessity. The human nervous system flourishes when it can rely on predictable patterns and deliberate pauses. Stable rituals soothe the brain, lower cortisol, reset circadian rhythms, allow melatonin to rise and ebb as it should. In this way, ritual is not just symbolic—it is structural, shaping the day's architecture, creating edges where once there was only the blur of endless scrolling. For those ground down by chronic stress or burnout, whose internal clocks are hijacked by adrenaline, such scaffolding is vital.

Perhaps the most transformative expression of sacred slowness is the ancient rhythm of weekly rest—the Sabbath, though not in any rigid or sectarian sense. Across the world's cultures, some version of a pause-day has existed: a counterweight to the demands of labour, a breathing space for the soul. In Jewish life, Shabbat begins with sunset, a deliberate turning away from the tyranny of the clock. In Hindu traditions, certain days are dedicated to puja, fasting, or silence, guided by the stars. Many Indigenous peoples have marked the pause with fire circles, storytelling, or time on the land. These were not quaint customs—they were technologies of the spirit, designed to fend off exhaustion of the heart.

In a secular frame, the Sabbath can take any form that breaks the cycle of constant output: a Sunday free from screens, a slow shared meal, an afternoon wandering outdoors. The shape matters less than the commitment. When the week holds a true, repeated stopping point, the psyche begins to shift. Monday no longer arrives as a thief in the night but as a companion after rest. Slowness ceases to be an escape and becomes part of the weave.

To re-sacralise time is also to reconsider the most ordinary acts. Sacredness is not a matter of aesthetic but of attitude. Combing one's hair with care, tidying a table with gratitude, preparing food without distraction—such acts become ceremonies when approached with attention. The difference between routine and ritual lies in the quality of presence. A morning oil massage can whisper safety to the body; five measured breaths before opening the inbox can remind the mind that presence outweighs performance. Over time, these micro-ceremonies form an internal rhythm resilient to the chaos beyond.

There is, too, a quietly radical edge to sacred slowness. To slow down in a culture that fetishises acceleration is an act of dissent. It refuses the logic that equates worth with output. It resists the erosion of boundaries between work and rest, the algorithmic capture of attention. Reclaiming time as sacred is not merely self-care—it is cultural resistance. It is a reminder that human beings are not machines, that wellness cannot be squeezed into tighter schedules. As Jenny Odell has written, in a world where attention is endlessly monetised, withholding it becomes one of the most subversive acts possible.

Still, the path back to slowness is not without its thorns. A nervous system addicted to urgency may rebel; stillness can feel unsettling, even dangerous. Silence sometimes unmasks grief, longing, or hollowness—and that is precisely where its medicine lies. Slowness exposes what speed hides. It creates room for integration, for joy to rise unforced, for intuition to speak without competing with the din. It is not indulgence but initiation, preparing body and mind alike for fuller presence.

Here, you will find ways back into this slower, truer time. You will encounter perspectives from traditions that see time not as a linear commodity but as a living relationship. You will see how rituals—whether inherited or newly crafted—can steady the mind and restore emotional continuity. You will be encouraged to build a modern Sabbath with boundaries firm enough to hold. And you may begin to notice the everyday thresholds—making tea, folding clothes, washing hands—not as drudgery, but as moments to return to yourself.

Sacred slowness is not a retreat from reality but a turning towards it: the breath, the body, the sky overhead. It is not anti-modern; it is deeply human. In a world that thrives on your distraction, your presence is your power. In a culture that counts your hours, your rhythm is your quiet sovereignty.

To slow down is not to be left behind. It is, perhaps for the first time, to arrive.

Time Isn't Money, It's Medicine:

Time, in the dominant economic imagination, is a resource to be spent, saved, maximised. We are trained to treat each hour like a coin to invest in productivity, its value tied to output. Calendars become battlegrounds. Hours become commodities. The day is carved into tasks, appointments, deadlines. From childhood, we are schooled in clock time—not to feel it, but to conquer it. This framing is not neutral. It shapes the nervous system, the psyche, the social order. And it carries a cost: not only exhaustion, but alienation from time's original essence—as a rhythm, a medicine, a teacher.

To say "time is money" is to collapse two profoundly different logics into one. Money is a tool of abstraction, transaction, control. Time, in contrast, is a field of relationship. It is cyclical, embodied, alive. In traditional cultures across continents—from the Vedic seers of ancient India to the land-tethered timekeepers of the Andes and the Yoruba—*time was not owned; it was observed.* It moved with the sun, the tides, the phases of the moon. It pulsed through breath, ritual, and season. To be well was to be in rhythm with it. To be ill, often, was to be out of sync.

What has been largely lost in modernity is not time itself, but *right relationship with time.* And this misalignment is more than conceptual—it is somatic. The body, governed by circadian, ultradian, and hormonal rhythms, is not designed for constant acceleration. When time is fractured—when the day is sliced into notifications and microtasks—the nervous system defaults to hypervigilance. Stress hormones surge. Digestion stalls. Sleep becomes shallow. This is not merely correlation. It is causation. *Time anxiety is a form of physiological disruption*—a silent epidemic in white-collar and caregiving professions alike.

Indigenous timekeeping systems offer a counterpoint—not as nostalgia, but as epistemological challenge. In many First Nations cultures, time is not linear but relational. The Lakota refer to "natural time" as something felt through the land's needs. The Andean Quechua speak of time as something that arrives from behind—not something one moves into, but something that moves through. In this sense, to heal one's relationship with time is not to manage it better, but to *enter into humility with it.* Time becomes not a tool for control, but a context for participation.

Vedic philosophy offers a parallel, highly sophisticated articulation. Rather than treating time as uniform and objective, it maps time across scales—micro (moment), meso (day), and macro (cosmic cycle). The concept of *kāla* (time) is deeply embedded in the Ayurvedic and yogic traditions—not just as a backdrop to human activity, but as a force of nature with dharmic implications. Specific times of day are considered energetically distinct. Morning is governed by *vāta* and is ideal for spiritual practice. Midday, ruled by *pitta*, supports digestion and activity. Evening, infused with *kapha*, invites rest and integration. This isn't superstition—it is a biological attunement refined over millennia.

Modern science, interestingly, is beginning to confirm what these systems long intuited. The field of chronobiology—particularly the work of Nobel Prize–winning researchers in circadian rhythm—has shown that the timing of light exposure, food intake, and movement significantly influences hormonal balance, immune function, and emotional resilience. One's body is not a machine; it is a clock with thousands of synchronised gears. And those gears turn best when time is experienced as *ritual*, not regimen.

Ritual, in this context, is not necessarily spiritual or performative. It is functional, grounding, adaptive. It gives the nervous system predictable markers in an unpredictable world. A cup of tea at 4 p.m. can anchor a person in the midst of chaos. A morning walk at sunrise can regulate serotonin and dopamine levels. A weekly day of rest—free of screens, tasks, or metrics—can recalibrate the entire endocrine system. *Ritual doesn't steal time; it gives time shape.*

One reason modern people fear slowing down is that they equate it with falling behind. But this assumes a race—and a finish line. The Vedic tradition offers another view: that time is not a ladder, but a wheel. One does not fall behind time; one falls out of resonance with it. Healing, then, involves entraining one's daily rhythms to time's larger intelligence. This is not inefficiency—it is ecological literacy. It is the art of aligning with nature's tempo rather than the algorithm's.

Even within the economic paradigm, cracks are forming. Scholars such as Jonathan Crary and academics within the "slow scholarship" movement have critiqued the 24/7 model of attention and output. The rise of burnout as a mainstream diagnosis has forced workplaces to confront the human cost of chronocapitalism. But institutional reform remains slow. What individuals can do—now—is begin to reclaim their internal time. To honour the body's need for pause. To stop wearing exhaustion as a badge. *To treat rest not as reward, but as rhythm.*

Real-world shifts are already underway. In Denmark, companies have experimented with "quiet hours" that ban internal meetings to protect focused work time. In Japan, where *karoshi* (death by overwork) remains a tragic reality, initiatives like "forest bathing" have been institutionalised as public health strategies. In India, the growing resurgence of *dinacharya* (daily rhythm) among urban wellness practitioners reflects a desire to return to natural cycles. And globally, there is a quiet movement of people rediscovering the Sabbath—not in religious dogma, but in digital abstinence, slow meals, and contemplative rituals.

Redefining time as medicine begins with language. To stop saying "I don't have time" and start saying "That's not aligned with my rhythm." To stop asking "How can I do more?" and begin asking "What does this moment need?" It continues with small, deliberate actions: lighting a candle at dusk, turning off notifications after dinner, carving out unscheduled space without guilt. It culminates in a shift of cosmology—from time as taskmaster to time as companion.

This reframing is not soft. It is revolutionary. Because when time becomes medicine, presence becomes priority. When time becomes sacred, the sacred returns to the day. And when the body remembers what it feels like to move in rhythm with the world, healing ceases to be a future goal—it becomes a present practice.

Rituals That Hold You Together:

Stability in modern life is rarely an external condition; it is more often an internal competence—one that must be cultivated with intent. As the outer world grows noisier, faster, and increasingly fragmented, our inner world requires stronger scaffolding. Not rigid routines that become new burdens, but subtle structures—micro-rituals—that tether attention, emotion, and presence. These are the invisible ligaments of daily wellbeing: small, repeating gestures that hold us together when everything else feels like it's coming apart.

In a culture that confuses discipline with productivity and ritual with religiosity, it's easy to overlook the emotional utility of ritualised action. Yet across traditions, micro-rituals have always functioned as more than habits. They are containers for consciousness. They bind psyche to soma, meaning to motion. From an Ayurvedic practitioner lighting a copper lamp at dawn to a Japanese tea host arranging cups with meditative precision, the action is not incidental—it is medicinal. The healing is in the rhythm. *Rituals are less about the thing you do and more about the way you do the thing.*

Neurologically, the repetition inherent in ritual helps regulate the autonomic nervous system. When performed regularly, even the most modest acts—anointing the body with warm oil, whispering a short prayer, sitting quietly before sleep—communicate safety to the brain. This is not symbolic; it is biochemical. The predictability of the act downregulates cortisol, supports vagal tone, and restores coherence between the sympathetic and parasympathetic systems. This is especially relevant in chronic stress states, where the body remains stuck in mobilisation or collapse. In such cases, a morning oil massage (*abhyanga*) is not just a wellness indulgence—it is a neurosensory intervention.

Micro-rituals also function as emotional bookmarks. They allow us to bracket time, to transition with intention. In a world where many move from emails to dinner to phone scrolling without pause, these rituals can serve as punctuation—allowing the psyche to catch its breath between chapters. A warm drink before work. A deep breath after meetings. A journal entry by candlelight at night. These are not aesthetic affectations. They are ways to metabolise the day, rather than accumulate it. *Without rituals of release, experience becomes residue.*

The psychological dimension of ritual lies in its power to create meaning. Clinical psychologist and grief researcher Robert Neimeyer has long argued that people do not simply suffer from trauma—they suffer from unintegrated meaning. Ritual becomes a technology for meaning-making. It provides a container through which to process events that defy logic. This is why nearly every culture has ritualised forms for birth, death, change, and healing. But what modernity often forgets is that *small transitions need containers too.* Leaving a job. Ending a relationship. Completing a project. These are thresholds. And thresholds require attention.

Even seemingly mundane micro-rituals can carry deep restorative power when practiced with intention. Consider the act of prayerful breathing: three slow inhalations, each paired with a phrase of gratitude or surrender. When repeated daily, the nervous system begins to associate the breath with safety. Or journaling: not as narrative therapy per se, but as a quiet reckoning with the self—asking, *What did I learn today? What do I need to release? What will I carry forward?* This is not about self-analysis. It is about self-anchoring.

The potency of a ritual does not lie in its complexity, but in its resonance. For some, this may mean applying sesame oil to the soles of the feet before bed—a practice known in Ayurveda to stabilise *vāta* and support deep sleep. For others, it may be placing a hand on the heart and whispering a name each morning—a loved one, an intention, a prayer. What matters is not orthodoxy but relationship. A ritual is medicine only if the body recognises it as such.

Clinical research is beginning to explore what ancient cultures have always known—that micro-rituals can modulate affective states and even immunological function. A 2020 study published in *Frontiers in Psychology* found that brief, intentional rituals performed daily had measurable impacts on emotional resilience and perceived stress levels. Participants who developed and adhered to their own "ritual design"—simple actions like lighting incense, reciting affirmations, or doing breathwork before meals—reported a greater sense of internal coherence and adaptability under pressure. This is not incidental. It points to ritual as a core tool of stress ecology.

There is also an ethical dimension to reclaiming ritual. In late capitalism, every hour is monetised, every habit scrutinised for optimisation. Micro-rituals offer resistance—not in protest, but in presence. They allow a person to declare, *This moment is mine. This body is not a machine. This act does not need to be efficient to be worthwhile.* That declaration is not trivial. It is subversive. Especially for those whose identities have been historically shaped by servitude, overfunctioning, or chronic caregiving, ritual becomes a form of reclamation. It says: I am not what I produce. I am what I attend to.

In trauma-informed somatic work, ritual often plays a foundational role in re-establishing a sense of safety in the body. Therapists may guide clients to create small daily rituals that ground attention in the here-and-now: placing a warm cloth over the face to soothe the vagus nerve, gently rocking in a chair, tracing the outline of one's hand while breathing. These may appear simple, but they speak directly to the limbic brain, which does not respond to logic, only felt safety. *When ritual is paired with attunement, it becomes a bridge from dissociation to embodiment.*

Yet, not all rituals are restorative. There is a distinction to be made between compulsive routines and nourishing rhythms. When ritual becomes rigid, performative, or laden with guilt, it loses its healing valence. The key differentiator is *attunement.* A ritual should feel like a return, not a performance. If it becomes a source of stress, it ceases to serve. The point is not to create a schedule of perfect self-care, but to establish rhythm within which one can be imperfect and still held.

To implement such rituals requires more than strategy—it requires permission. Permission to slow down. To prioritise what cannot be measured. To attend to the invisible architecture of wellbeing. This is where the shift must occur—not from busyness to slowness alone, but from *disconnection to coherence.* Micro-rituals are not aesthetic lifestyle hacks. They are gestures of continuity in a fractured world. They are reminders that even amidst uncertainty, one can still choose rhythm over reaction.

Ultimately, the rituals that hold us together are not grand or ceremonial. They are quiet. Repetitive. Often unnoticed by others. But over time, they become encoded in the nervous system as safety. In the psyche as meaning. In the heart as refuge. And it is precisely these ordinary actions—performed with extraordinary care—that allow a person not only to survive stress, but to digest it, metabolise it, and return to wholeness.

Weekly Recalibration:

To pause—deliberately, unapologetically—is not merely to rest. It is to defy a cultural operating system that defines value by velocity and output. In modern life, where the weekend has been colonised by backlog and leisure repackaged as content creation, the idea of a Sabbath—a full-bodied weekly rest—can seem archaic, even indulgent. Yet it is precisely this kind of rhythmic stillness that many nervous systems now require for survival. The need is not moral or religious. It is physiological, psychological, and existential. A weekly recalibration, properly understood, is not a luxury. It is essential hygiene for the mind and body.

The ancient Hebrew Sabbath offered a radical principle: that even the act of creation must yield to cessation. The world, in this telling, was not completed in six days, but in seven—because the seventh was not a void, but a form. Rest was not an interruption of work; it was a category of being. This orientation is echoed across indigenous, Taoist, and Vedic time traditions, where life is measured not only in tasks completed, but in cycles honoured. These systems encode a different intelligence: *Time does not belong to us to spend; we belong to it, and must keep its rhythm.*

Contrast this with the dominant modern conception of time: extractive, linear, and monetised. The logic of productivity culture has recast every hour as a resource to optimise, every weekend as deferred labour. This shift has profound implications for stress physiology. Without recurring, intentional recovery windows, the stress-response system remains hypertonic—locked in patterns of vigilance, over-effort, and adrenal depletion. Weekly recalibration becomes not only a countercultural act but a neurological imperative.

What makes the modern Sabbath different from its historical precedents is that it must often be reclaimed rather than inherited. For most readers, there is no inherited blueprint. There is no built-in infrastructure. Instead, the Sabbath must be consciously designed: a recurring 24-hour period that is protected from obligation, from digital intrusion, and from the imperative to improve, upgrade, or monetise. It is a space in which the nervous system, the mind, and the psyche are allowed to soften back into their natural intelligence—beyond performance, beyond urgency.

This is not about dogmatic withdrawal. Nor is it about performative wellness. The modern Sabbath must adapt to complex lives and multiple responsibilities. What matters is not aesthetic purity, but energetic shift. The Sabbath recalibrates not because of what one avoids, but because of what one attends to: unstructured time, slowness, nature, real conversation, food prepared without rush, music without agenda, time spent without tracking. The recalibration happens through presence. *Sabbath is less about rest and more about remembering what it feels like to be unhurried and whole.*

Cross-cultural practices of rest offer models, not mandates. In West African spiritual lineages, market days double as sacred time—not merely for commerce, but for music, exchange, and embodied rest. Among the Māori of Aotearoa, *noho tahi* (sitting together) is a communal mode of rest that prioritises relational energy over isolation. In Japanese culture, the concept of *ma*—a pause or emptiness that gives shape to experience—can be expressed in ritualised tea-making or shared silence. Each tradition encodes the same insight: *True rest is not passive, it is participatory.* It involves tuning in, not dropping out.

Modern neuroscience confirms what these traditions have always intuited. Regular rest—particularly in the form of intentional downregulation—restores executive function, modulates immune response, and enhances memory consolidation. But the benefits go deeper than metrics. Weekly recalibration allows for the integration of experience. Without pause, life becomes a continuous feed; we accumulate events without digesting them. Rest, properly structured, is not a break from meaning—it is what makes meaning metabolically possible.

The spiritual dimension of a weekly Sabbath is not necessarily religious. It is reverent. The pause becomes a ceremony of remembrance: *I am not here to serve the machine.* That remembrance is radical in systems that ask us to monetise our identities, to always be available, to compete with our own previous selves. The modern Sabbath is not about rejecting technology, but about choosing sovereignty over it. It says: today, I will not be surveilled by the glow of devices. I will not outsource attention to an algorithm. I will not measure my worth in what I produce.

There are tensions to navigate. For caregivers, shift workers, or anyone operating within structural inequities, the idea of a protected day off can feel out of reach. This is not a failure of the Sabbath—it is an indictment of the systems that erode access to it. In this context, recalibration may require adaptation: half-days, structured evenings, collective pauses organised with others. The spirit remains the same: to reclaim time from extraction and reframe it as medicine. The point is not to replicate ancient rest structures but to apply their wisdom to modern conditions.

Ritual can support this process. Lighting a specific candle, turning off devices at a designated time, opening a text that is read only on that day—these actions can help demarcate the transition into sacred time. They help the body shift gears, to know that *this time is different.* Some may begin their Sabbath with a shared meal, a nature walk, or a period of silence. Others may anchor it through breathwork, music, or journaling. What matters is that the act be repeated—not as obligation, but as orientation. Ritual is not performance; it is punctuation.

Importantly, recalibration is not just about rest—it is about re-alignment. It invites inquiry: What have I become entangled in? Where have I overcommitted? What needs to be let go? The Sabbath becomes a mirror held up to the week. It reveals what is essential and what is inherited. It clarifies priorities. It provides space for grief, for gratitude, for the kind of integration that cannot happen while multitasking. This is how rest becomes generative: not the absence of doing, but the reconstitution of being.

For those living with chronic stress or recovering from burnout, weekly recalibration is not optional. It is a cornerstone of healing. Without regular intervals of nervous system downregulation, the stress physiology becomes self-perpetuating. Adrenal fatigue, sleep disruption, hormonal imbalance, cognitive fog—all are exacerbated by the absence of cyclical rest. The Sabbath is a way of saying to the body: *You are safe enough to release now.* This invitation is not made through thought, but through structure. Through action.

Ultimately, a weekly Sabbath is not just a personal practice—it is a collective intervention. When rest is reclaimed, so too is humanity. The ripple effects extend outward: families relate differently, decisions are made more wisely, communities begin to recalibrate around rhythms that serve rather than extract. Rest is not a reward for productivity. It is a form of protest against a worldview that measures time only in transactions. It is a sanctuary where nothing needs to be earned.

The modern Sabbath will not resemble its historical counterpart in form—but it can in function. Whether observed on a Sunday, a Tuesday, or a sequence of smaller intervals, its essence is the same: *Pause. Recollect. Reinhabit.* Not to escape life, but to re-enter it with more discernment, more coherence, and more space to choose who we are becoming.

Ceremony for the Everyday:

Ceremony, in its most vital form, is not reserved for sacred buildings or milestone events. It belongs in the quiet folds of ordinary life. Yet modernity has distanced ritual from the everyday. What was once woven into the fabric of daily tasks has been exiled to the margins—replaced by efficiency, speed, and hyper-functionality. In this cultural climate, making tea is merely hydration. Walking is transport. Cleaning is a chore. The soul of the action—the presence, the pattern, the reverence—gets stripped away. To reclaim the ceremonial in everyday life is not sentimentalism. It is a sophisticated act of nervous system repair, cultural resistance, and personal coherence.

What does it mean to make tea as a ceremony, not a task? Consider the Japanese *chado*, or "Way of Tea"—a tradition that transforms the making and serving of tea into an act of aesthetic, ethical, and spiritual significance. In this context, tea is not a beverage but a medium through which attentiveness, grace, and humility are practised. There is silence between gestures. There is a sequence that matters. Every part of the process—the pouring of water, the folding of a cloth—reorients the participant from speed to precision, from distraction to intimacy. The ceremony does not occur *during* tea. It *is* tea.

Of course, most lives do not accommodate a full *chado*. But the insight endures: *ritual is a way of elevating the mundane to the meaningful.* When we infuse daily acts with rhythm, intention, and care, we activate a part of the psyche that recognises beauty, connection, and belonging. This doesn't require elaborate tools or spiritual paraphernalia. It requires orientation. The difference between brushing your teeth and *marking the end of the day* is not in the act but in the awareness. The same applies to cooking, washing, stretching, sweeping. These acts become healing not through change in content, but through change in consciousness.

This reorientation is not abstract. It has measurable consequences for psychological wellbeing and autonomic balance. Neuroscientific studies have shown that repetitive, embodied actions—particularly when done with focused attention—help regulate the vagus nerve, which plays a central role in modulating stress responses. This explains why monks in nearly every contemplative tradition perform simple, repetitive chores as part of their spiritual training: not in spite of their simplicity, but *because* of it. The rhythm of the broom on the floor, or the cloth on the table, becomes a form of prayer—one that speaks in the language of the body.

Modern trauma therapy echoes this. In somatic and polyvagal approaches, repeated sensory rituals—hand-washing, grounding breaths, holding warm cups—are deployed as tools for stabilisation. These are not metaphysical gestures; they are practical interventions that help the body feel safe enough to inhabit the present moment. The ceremonial lens, when applied to daily life, offers a non-verbal form of self-attunement. It teaches the nervous system: you are allowed to slow down. You are allowed to feel. You are allowed to be here without defending yourself.

Cleaning, in this light, is no longer a means to an end but a form of restoration. In Zen monasteries, the act of cleaning is as sacred as meditation—both function to clear residue, physical and psychic. The same ethos can be applied to the domestic sphere. When sweeping the floor is done with mindfulness, it becomes a release of stale energy. When dishes are washed slowly, with warm water and breath awareness, they serve as a mirror for internal clarity. This isn't romanticism—it's energetics. When we relate to our environment with presence, the boundary between inner and outer life begins to dissolve. The room becomes an extension of the body. The act becomes an offering.

This orientation doesn't require perfection. If ceremony is rigid or performative, it defeats its purpose. The power of everyday ritual lies in its informality. A brief pause before drinking water. A hand on the chest after waking. A short exhale before speaking. These micro-ceremonies punctuate the day with awareness. They are not about control but coherence. They interrupt the automation of living and invite the return of agency. And that is where healing begins—not with dramatic interventions, but with the smallest acts reclaimed.

Walking, too, is a potent site of transformation when approached ceremonially. Not for steps counted or calories burned, but as a form of embodied presence. Indigenous traditions have long regarded walking as a dialogue with the land—a way of remembering one's place in the web of life. In Taoist thought, walking meditation aligns breath, step, and attention to create inner harmony. A daily walk, taken without devices, without urgency, without agenda, becomes a corridor back to oneself. The world is re-encountered not as something to rush through, but as something to relate to.

The Western wellness industry often packages ritual as aesthetic—candles, oils, bowls, feathers. But true ceremony requires no props. Its power lies in rhythm, repetition, and meaning. A breath repeated the same way every morning can be a more effective ritual than any curated toolkit. What the nervous system longs for is not stimulation, but predictability. Ceremony provides that—not as monotony, but as safety. Repetition becomes a holding structure. It says: *This moment is known. You are not lost. There is order here.*

Critically, ceremony must be decoupled from performance. It is not something one does for social media, for validation, or even for self-improvement. Ceremony is not a technique—it is a relationship. When small acts are infused with respect and rhythm, they return us to right relationship with time, body, place, and process. This is where stress resilience is built: not in avoiding challenge, but in cultivating coherence amidst it.

There is also an ethical dimension. By slowing down and reclaiming presence, we begin to participate differently in the world. Consumption becomes more conscious. Relationships become less transactional. Even speech begins to shift—less reaction, more reflection. This re-patterning of daily life is not separate from broader healing; it *is* the work. The ceremonies we enact shape the consciousness we inhabit.

There is a growing movement toward slow living, but unless slowness is anchored in ritual, it risks becoming another aspirational aesthetic. True ceremonial living is not about pace alone—it is about presence. It asks not how slowly you are moving, but *how deeply you are attending.* This is what turns mundane routines into medicinal rituals. It is what allows the ordinary to become extraordinary—not in appearance, but in impact.

When we reclaim small acts as ceremony, we dismantle the binary between sacred and secular. We remind ourselves that healing is not something that occurs at retreats or only in crisis. It happens while slicing fruit, folding clothes, boiling rice. It happens when we stop waiting for special occasions and begin treating every occasion as worthy of attention. In a culture addicted to novelty, ceremony is revolutionary precisely because it honours repetition. It says: this again, and again, and again—with care.

Ultimately, ceremony for the everyday teaches a different mode of being—one that values depth over speed, attention over output, sufficiency over spectacle. It is a mode that restores not only the nervous system, but the soul. And the best part? It is available now, without needing to buy, fix, or become anything else. It begins where you are, with what you have, in the next small act you choose to honour.

Chapter 9
Healing in Relationship

For decades now, the conversation about stress has been anchored in a strangely persistent myth: that the individual stands alone, sovereign over their mental state, responsible for both the cause and cure of their distress. We are told that stress springs from faulty decisions, weak coping strategies, or some quirk of brain chemistry—and, conveniently, that the remedy lies in personal effort: download a mindfulness app, master a breathing technique, keep a gratitude journal, adjust your diet. It is a tidy story. It is also misleading. Such a framing strips stress of its social, historical, and structural roots, reducing it to a chemical glitch inside a single body. Yet stress, in truth, is not merely biochemical. It is a social flare, a fracture in relationship, a reflex to disconnection, inequality, and the looming shadow of systemic threat. This chapter asks you to consider a different premise: that healing is not a solitary endeavour, but a relational, collective—indeed, often political—act.

A substantial and still-growing body of work in neurobiology, attachment theory, and trauma research affirms something ancient cultures have long understood: the human nervous system cannot restore itself in isolation. We are designed—wired, quite literally—for co-regulation, that delicate, often unconscious process where our emotional states find balance through attuned connection with others. Safety, in this light, is not an individual conquest but a shared condition. A calm voice, the grounded steadiness of someone nearby, a meeting of eyes that says without words, "I see you"—these are not optional niceties. They are the stuff of medicine.

If we accept this, the consequences are not small. Mental health ceases to be purely the territory of the individual psyche. Strategies that ignore the wider social landscape will, by their nature, falter. Healing spaces must elevate relational intelligence alongside technique. Practitioners—therapists, coaches, clinicians—are called to examine the power structures implicit in their roles. The healer is not a heroic saviour swooping in to correct a flawed life, but a steady presence who walks alongside, bearing witness and co-creating safety.

We begin, then, with a dismantling of the hyper-individualism that saturates today's wellness industry. Colonial legacies, capitalist logic, and medical reductionism have all, in their way, warped our sense of what stress and healing truly are. To define trauma purely as a personal pathology is to overlook the bodily imprints of systemic racism, entrenched poverty, or the erasure of culture. Where suffering is rooted in collective harm, the solution cannot be confined to the individual. The wound must be understood within its broader ecology.

Consider the lived reality of racialised stress. A Black woman navigating daily microaggressions in a white-majority workplace may present with signs akin to anxiety—hypervigilance, exhaustion, an emotional guardedness. But these are not flaws in her coping system. They are intelligent, adaptive responses to an unsafe relational environment. The work of healing, for her, lies not in "repairing" thought patterns or calming physiology in isolation, but in transforming the relational field—through affirming community, cultural anchoring, and structural change. To label this solely as a mental health issue is to miss its essential truth.

It is in this light that we see the enduring wisdom of traditional healing systems. In many Indigenous, African, and Asian worldviews, health is not measured by individual stability but by the integrity of relationships—between person and community, the living and the ancestral, people and land. Illness signals rupture, and healing is enacted through reconnection. Western models, conversely, have pathologised dependence and exalted autonomy. Yet autonomy, without connection, is a hollow prize. Our nervous systems are not built for self-sufficiency; they are calibrated through interdependence.

This understanding shifts the therapeutic emphasis from method to presence. Clients rarely heal because a practitioner selects precisely the right technique from a manual. They heal when they are profoundly "felt"—when the other person's nervous system offers a steady rhythm of attunement, containment, acceptance. That is co-regulation in action. And its relevance extends far beyond therapy rooms. In families, workplaces, circles of friends, faith communities—everywhere—we serve as barometers for one another's emotional climate. One steady, regulated person can alter the atmosphere for an entire group. This is no poetic flourish. It is physiology.

The ripple effects are considerable. If stress is, at its root, relational, then healing must involve mending the web of relationship. This means not only repairing interpersonal bonds but re-establishing ties to cultural identity, spiritual tradition, and communal rhythms. In such spaces, belonging ceases to be a gentle abstraction and becomes an active intervention. When people are embedded in environments that affirm who they are and honour their dignity, measurable biological shifts occur: cortisol levels ease, heart rate variability improves, chronic inflammation diminishes. No pill, no cognitive drill, can replicate the potency of being genuinely welcomed.

Ritual, too, takes on a new clarity. Collective practices—be they ancestral rites, shared meals, or gatherings for grief—do more than mark time. They restore coherence to the group body. They tell the nervous system, in a language older than words: you are not alone; you are woven into a pattern. In an age that prizes speed, spectacle, and performance, ritual slows us down, grounds us, and reminds us that no one was built to bear the weight of life in isolation.

This is not, to be clear, a dismissal of personal agency or inner work. It is a matter of context. You may meditate faithfully, keep a meticulous journal, regulate your breath with discipline—but if you step back into a setting of chronic relational threat, your gains will erode. Safety is a collaborative creation. The nervous system must feel—not merely think—that it is not abandoned. This explains why trauma recovery so often accelerates when someone finds their "chosen family" or a group that mirrors back their worth. The gaze of an attuned other can rewrite what solitude could never touch.

There is also a caution here for those in healing roles. The romanticised healer archetype, with its undertones of rescue and expertise, can quietly undermine the client's sense of self. In a relational frame, the practitioner is not an elevated authority but an equal participant. This dismantles the saviour dynamic and affirms the innate capacity of the person seeking help. It also shields practitioners from burnout, releasing them from the unsustainable burden of being solely responsible for change.

Yet we cannot ignore the societal scaffolding around all this. Deep, attuned connection demands time, presence, and a freedom from certain pressures—resources that many lack. In cultures driven by productivity and saturated with digital noise, relational health can feel out of reach. This forces us into political territory: what structures make true connection possible? How might schools, workplaces, healthcare systems be redesigned to sustain relational wellbeing rather than merely individual efficiency? There is no simple blueprint, but the necessity is plain: if stress is a social illness, healing requires social vision.

Here, then, the chapter offers both the conceptual and the practical: the neuroscience underpinning co-regulation, exercises to nurture relational safety, approaches to dissolve healer-hero hierarchies, and real-world stories of belonging as a therapeutic force. Above all, it leaves you with a reoriented map—one where connection, not correction, sits at the centre of the healing process. In this age of widespread disconnection, such a map is more than a sentimental ideal. It is, quite simply, a survival plan. And one grounded, despite everything, in hope.

Stress as a Social Disease:

Stress has been domesticated into an individual story—something that happens inside the head, something to be managed through better breathing, stronger boundaries, or a more efficient calendar. Yet the origins of chronic stress do not arise in a vacuum. They often begin long before a person is born and stretch far beyond the walls of their home or office. Stress is not merely personal; it is social, historical, and structural. To frame stress solely as a private pathology is not just incomplete—it is a distortion that obscures its most powerful roots and, therefore, its most meaningful remedies.

When we localise stress in the individual, we imply that healing is a matter of personal competence. The anxious executive must learn to "manage" their stress through better self-discipline. The overwhelmed mother must simply "prioritise self-care." But this framing conceals a vital truth: *many forms of modern stress are entirely rational responses to environments that are chronically dysregulating.* The problem is not always inside the person—it is often the world around them. And to pretend otherwise is to gaslight both the nervous system and the person inhabiting it.

Take poverty as an example. A child growing up in an economically precarious household is likely to show elevated cortisol levels, increased vigilance, and behavioural agitation. These are not signs of internal dysfunction. They are adaptive, intelligent responses to uncertainty. Similarly, an adult navigating racial discrimination may exhibit symptoms that are clinically labelled as "generalised anxiety," when in fact these reactions are the residue of ongoing social threat. *When stress is chronic, it often reflects chronic conditions.* And when those conditions are shared by entire communities or generations, we are no longer in the realm of individual pathology—we are in the realm of social disease.

The term "social disease" is not hyperbolic. It points to the ways in which structures—economic systems, social hierarchies, political violence—embed themselves into biology. This is not metaphor; it is measurable. The field of epigenetics has demonstrated that trauma, malnutrition, and toxic stress can alter gene expression and be passed through generations. Studies of Holocaust survivors, Indigenous populations, and children of war have all shown a lingering imprint of historical trauma in both mental and physical health outcomes. *Ancestral pain is not symbolic—it is physiological.*

Yet mainstream approaches to stress often erase this context. Diagnostic manuals rarely reference systemic racism, displacement, or community disintegration as contributing factors. Instead, the focus is on the individual's coping style, emotional regulation, or cognitive distortions. While these lenses can be helpful, they are dangerously insufficient when they ignore the societal ecosystems people are forced to survive in. A therapy model that centres only the individual, while overlooking the collective, can inadvertently reinforce the very stress it claims to treat—by turning systemic wounds into personal failings.

This is especially true when we look at intergenerational trauma. Consider communities affected by colonisation: Indigenous groups whose land was taken, languages forbidden, spiritual practices criminalised. The grief of these ruptures did not vanish with time; it was metabolised into the psyche and physiology of descendants. Increased rates of addiction, violence, and mental illness in such communities are not moral defects or psychological weaknesses—they are expressions of inherited rupture. *The body remembers what history forgets.* And yet, when members of these communities seek help, they are often treated without any reference to that history.

It is equally urgent to consider the social nature of stress in modern urban environments. The disintegration of kinship structures, the fragmentation of neighbourhoods, and the omnipresence of digital surveillance have created a cultural ecology where many people feel chronically unsafe. The stress of modern life is often less about acute danger and more about persistent disconnection. *Hyper-individualism is not just a philosophical stance—it is a somatic wound.* We are social mammals, wired for mutual regulation, yet we are increasingly forced to navigate life as if we were sovereign units. The price of that illusion is exhaustion.

This understanding also demands a shift in the way we measure resilience. In the dominant model, resilience is the individual's capacity to bounce back from adversity. But what if resilience is not a trait, but a relationship? In collectivist cultures, resilience often emerges not from internal grit but from communal cohesion—from the knowledge that one is held by a larger whole. Mutual aid, extended family networks, and spiritual community are buffers against stress not because they remove adversity, but because they make it *bearable.* When support is embedded into the structure of daily life, stress does not disappear—but it does not have to metastasise into trauma.

Western psychology has only recently begun to catch up to what many Indigenous, African, and Asian traditions have long maintained: healing is not about the individual retreating into themselves; it is about returning to relationship—relationship with others, with land, with lineage, with spirit. This is not an abstract sentiment. It is a neurobiological imperative. Humans co-regulate through presence, voice tone, facial expression, shared ritual. The nervous system calibrates itself in relationship, not in isolation. And when those relationships are threatened, disrupted, or absent, stress is not just likely—it is inevitable.

From a public health perspective, this reconceptualisation has profound implications. If stress is socially constructed, then healing must also be socially designed. That means rethinking not only therapy but policy. Urban planning, labour rights, education reform—these are all domains of stress intervention. The built environment affects cortisol levels. Workplace culture affects immune function. Access to green space, clean air, and affordable housing are not luxuries—they are nervous system supports. To create a less stressed society, we must design a more relational world.

Even the language of stress management requires revision. To "manage" stress suggests that it is a resource to be scheduled, a defect to be corrected, or an enemy to be subdued. But stress, viewed from a social lens, is often the body's honest protest against relational breakdown. It is the physiological echo of unmet needs—for safety, for belonging, for dignity. Rather than managing stress, we might learn to *listen* to it—not as an irritant, but as an oracle. What if chronic stress is not a personal failure, but a social signal—a call to reconfigure how we live together?

For practitioners, this lens offers both a challenge and an invitation. It challenges the tendency to over-focus on internal dynamics at the expense of social realities. But it also opens the door to richer, more integrated practice. A trauma-informed approach cannot stop at somatic interventions. It must engage with cultural humility, historical literacy, and structural awareness. Healing is not neutral. It takes place within a moral and political landscape. To help someone truly heal, one must be willing to see what their body is reacting to—and that often means looking beyond the individual story.

As this chapter unfolds, the aim is not to discard individual approaches, but to expand them. Cognitive strategies, mindfulness practices, and somatic therapies remain valuable—but only when contextualised within the broader tapestry of social and ancestral forces. The hyper-individualistic frame must be softened, not because it is entirely wrong, but because it is fatally narrow. When we widen our view, we discover that stress is not just a private matter—it is a public health concern, a cultural inheritance, and a political challenge. And when we begin to treat it as such, new possibilities for relief, resilience, and repair begin to emerge.

Co-Regulation as the First Medicine:

Safety is not a thought—it's a felt sense, and one that is seldom achieved in solitude. While modern wellness culture often exhorts us to self-soothe, self-regulate, and develop inner resilience, neuroscience tells a more ancient truth: *the human nervous system is co-authored in relationship*. Long before we could walk or speak, we were learning to feel safe or unsafe through the gaze, tone, and touch of others. Co-regulation—this primal, physiological tuning between beings—is not a luxury of secure attachment; it is the foundation of all emotional healing.

To frame co-regulation as the first medicine is not metaphorical. The nervous system is a social organ, evolved to detect and respond to signals of safety or threat in other bodies. When someone breathes slowly beside us, when their eyes soften with compassion, when their voice carries warmth and steadiness—our body recognises the cues. The vagus nerve, responsible for parasympathetic calm, is deeply attuned to relational context. We may try to think ourselves into ease, but no amount of cognitive reframing can match the speed and potency of a regulated presence.

Polyvagal theory, developed by Dr Stephen Porges, offers a scientific framework for understanding this process. It describes how the autonomic nervous system is constantly scanning the environment through what he calls "neuroception"—an unconscious assessment of safety or danger. Importantly, neuroception does not rely on facts; it responds to cues. A person may be intellectually aware that they're not under threat, but if their environment is loud, chaotic, or emotionally cold, their nervous system will react defensively. This is why healing cannot be exclusively internal. *We don't just need safe thoughts—we need safe others.*

This is especially relevant in the context of chronic stress, trauma, and burnout. Many individuals experiencing dysregulation have learned to override their relational instincts, either because safe others were not available, or because connection itself became a source of threat. In such cases, the invitation to co-regulate may feel foreign or even suspicious. Yet it remains vital. A body that has been hurt in relationship often needs to *heal* in relationship. And not in grand gestures, but in the micro-moments: a breath mirrored, a silence held, a gaze that does not turn away.

The failure to recognise this truth has led to a proliferation of healing models that are disproportionately internalised and hyper-independent. Meditation apps, journaling practices, gratitude exercises—while beneficial, these strategies often presume the presence of an already-coherent self who can self-soothe at will. But what of those whose very sense of self was never fully formed in safety? What of those whose earliest environments taught them to brace rather than rest? For these individuals, inner work is important—but insufficient. *They need co-regulators before they can become self-regulators.*

In therapeutic settings, this shifts the role of the practitioner from fixer to anchor. The most transformative interventions are not always techniques—they are nervous system states. A clinician who can remain grounded in the face of a client's chaos offers something profound: not just insight, but a new relational template. As psychiatrist Dan Siegel puts it, "integration happens in the context of attuned relationships." It is not the words we say but the way we are that often determines whether healing unfolds.

Outside of therapy, co-regulation plays out in a thousand unnoticed interactions. The way a teacher pauses to validate a student's distress. The way a partner holds silence instead of fixing. The way friends synchronise laughter. These are not trivial moments—they are *medicine in motion.* Communities that lack access to traditional mental health services often rely heavily on these relational rituals. The shared meal, the communal prayer, the familial embrace—these are nervous system technologies, developed long before the invention of psychology.

Of course, co-regulation can also misfire. Just as safety is contagious, so is anxiety. Anyone who has sat in a tense room or lived with a chronically dysregulated parent knows this viscerally. The presence of another does not automatically soothe—it depends on that person's own internal coherence. This is why responsibility must accompany relational healing. If we wish to co-regulate effectively, we must tend to our own regulation first. Not perfectly, but with honesty and intention. *To be a calming presence, we must first become present to ourselves.*

There is also a social justice dimension to co-regulation that is often overlooked. Marginalised communities face chronic nervous system disruption not just from interpersonal trauma, but from systemic injustice. Racial profiling, transphobic policies, poverty, surveillance—these are not merely political issues, but somatic ones. When someone is told, through word or structure, that their body is not safe in public, their nervous system adapts accordingly. Healing in such contexts cannot be apolitical. It must involve creating environments—schools, workplaces, clinics—where safety is structurally and relationally embedded.

Practices that foster co-regulation do not require specialised training or therapeutic contexts. What they do require is presence, slowness, and attention to subtlety. Here are a few relational habits that deepen co-regulation, offered not as prescriptions but as possibilities:

– *Shared breathing*: Sit beside someone in silence and allow your breath to synchronise. No words. Just presence.
– *Vocal tone awareness*: Speak with intentional warmth and rhythm. Your tone carries more regulatory power than your content.
– *Facial softness*: Make eye contact that is gentle, not penetrating. A relaxed face is a signal of welcome.
– *Stillness and pacing*: Resist the impulse to fill silence. Let calmness accumulate in the pauses.

While these practices may sound simple, they are countercultural in a world obsessed with speed, productivity, and performance. Co-regulation is an antidote to all of that. It is not fast. It is not efficient. It cannot be gamified or optimised. It requires us to be fully human, in all our breath and body and slowness. And in that humanity lies the healing.

The implications of this are profound for every layer of society. In education, teachers who understand co-regulation can create classrooms that are not only more humane, but more effective. In medicine, clinicians who treat patients with attuned presence—not just prescriptions—can accelerate recovery in ways no drug alone can. In family life, parents who learn to regulate themselves before responding to a child's outburst can raise more resilient children. And in activism, communities that practice mutual regulation can sustain resistance without burnout.

To co-regulate is to remember that healing is relational. Not just because we feel better around calm people, but because *our biology depends on them.* We are not sealed containers. We are tuning forks. What we absorb and what we transmit determines the emotional climate of every room we enter. This does not mean we are responsible for other people's healing. But it does mean we are never neutral. We are either amplifying stress—or diffusing it.

As we come to reframe stress not merely as an individual fault line but as a social feedback loop, the case for co-regulation becomes clearer. It is not an optional skill or soft add-on. It is foundational. And it begins with a shift in posture: from managing others to meeting them, from analysing emotion to attuning to it, from fixing to *feeling with.* This is not sentiment—it is science. It is not a regression to dependency—it is a recognition of interdependence. Co-regulation is not the opposite of strength. It is the condition in which true resilience is born.

The Healer Is Not a Hero:

The cultural ideal of the healer as a hero—a saviour armed with wisdom, tools, and singular insight—is not merely outdated. It is actively harmful. It distorts the power dynamics of care, misrepresents the nature of healing, and burdens practitioners with an impossible expectation: to be the source of another's transformation. This archetype, long romanticised across medicine, psychology, and wellness, elevates the practitioner while often silencing the agency of the client or patient. The result is not empowerment but dependence, not liberation but hierarchy.

At the root of this distortion is a misreading of what healing is. Healing is not something one person gives to another. It is a co-emergent process, an unfolding that takes place within and between people. The healer does not deliver wholeness—they *accompany its reawakening.* Any practitioner who confuses their role as one of fixing, curing, or enlightening risks interfering with the very intelligence they are meant to support. *To overstep is to disempower.*

The origins of the healer-as-hero myth lie in both historical and psychological dynamics. From the tribal shaman to the modern surgeon, the image of the healer as a figure of authority has been central to many societies. In contexts of survival—pandemics, trauma, spiritual crisis—this elevation made sense. Expertise was needed, trust was critical, and decisive action saved lives. But in the long arc of care, especially with chronic stress and emotional pain, heroism becomes an obstacle. Chronic healing is not about decisive intervention. It is about *sustained presence* and *relational depth.*

What many clients need is not rescue, but respectful witnessing. The act of being deeply seen, heard, and felt—without being pathologised or corrected—is inherently therapeutic. This does not negate the need for knowledge or skill. It reframes their purpose. Techniques, modalities, and insights are tools. But *the practitioner is not the tool.* They are a co-regulator, a co-inquirer, a companion. Their value lies less in what they do, and more in *how they are*—attuned, transparent, and ethically bound to shared humanity.

Nowhere is this more evident than in trauma work. Survivors of trauma often carry not only physical and psychological wounds, but relational wounds—those inflicted by neglect, betrayal, and power abuse. When a practitioner unconsciously positions themselves as the expert who knows better, who defines the problem and prescribes the path, they risk reenacting the very dynamics that caused harm. Safety, in such cases, is not achieved through competence alone. It is created through humility, responsiveness, and *an ethos of collaboration.*

Contemporary neuroscience supports this shift. Research into the social nervous system reveals that healing is less about information transfer and more about *neurobiological synchrony.* The practitioner's regulated state influences the client's system far more than any verbal technique. Polyvagal-informed clinicians understand this: the tone of voice, rhythm of speech, quality of gaze, and openness of posture communicate more than credentials ever could. When a client feels met rather than managed, the conditions for self-repair emerge organically.

But what sustains the hero dynamic, despite all this evidence? Partly, it is institutional. Medical training, psychotherapy schools, and even alternative healing certifications often reinforce hierarchical structures. Practitioners are taught to diagnose, treat, and lead. Less attention is paid to relational intelligence, power awareness, or co-creation. Furthermore, clients—especially those raised in authority-based systems—may themselves seek out the hero figure. It feels safer, more efficient. Tell me what's wrong. Tell me what to do. Fix me.

This creates a feedback loop of dependency: the practitioner feels needed, the client feels temporarily held, and the deeper work of self-trust remains untouched. Breaking this cycle requires courage on both sides. The practitioner must risk relinquishing their pedestal. The client must risk stepping into their own authority. This is not always comfortable. But it is essential for sustainable healing. *No one can grow inside a power imbalance.*

There are, of course, nuances. There are moments when directive care is appropriate—during acute crises, medical emergencies, or early-stage containment in trauma work. But these moments are not the whole. And they must always be followed by restoration of agency. The measure of a good practitioner is not how many answers they have, but *how they support others in discovering their own.* This is not a diminishment of the role. It is a maturation.

The shift from healer-as-hero to healer-as-partner has broad implications for professional ethics. It requires a redefinition of boundaries—not to distance, but to dignify. Boundaries are not walls; they are agreements about respect. In a partnership model, the practitioner is transparent about their scope, fallibility, and process. They do not pretend to be beyond projection, but they *stay in conscious relationship with it.* They do not deny transference—they navigate it with care. The client is not idealised, infantilised, or fixed. They are engaged as a sovereign being.

Some of the most promising approaches in contemporary healing embrace this ethos. Narrative therapy, for example, rejects the pathology-based model and positions the client as the author of their own life. The therapist becomes a curious collaborator, asking questions that open space rather than prescribing solutions. Similarly, somatic practices such as Hakomi or Focusing do not impose insight but invite *felt sensing*—trusting the body's intelligence rather than the therapist's theory.

Indigenous and community-based healing systems have long modelled these principles. In many traditions, the healer is not a separate class of person, but a role held temporarily, with responsibility to the collective. Their power comes not from superiority, but from service. They are not asked to be perfect—they are asked to be honest, relational, and in right relation with the unseen. This cultural framing prevents the inflation and burnout so common in Western practitioner roles. *When healing is shared, so is the burden.*

It is also worth noting that the healer-as-hero myth fuels practitioner burnout. Those who carry the unspoken expectation of transformation—for every client, in every session—are bound to collapse under the weight. They cannot grieve the inevitable limits of their role, nor celebrate the quiet power of non-intervention. When practitioners reframe themselves as participants rather than providers, their work becomes more sustainable. They can be present without pressure, responsible without rescuing, effective without ego.

Perhaps the most radical act a healer can do is not to heal, but to *hold space for healing to arise.* This may mean asking fewer questions, allowing longer silences, honouring the client's defences rather than challenging them, or simply naming what is true: "I don't have an answer, but I'm here with you." These are not acts of weakness. They are acts of trust—in the client, in the process, and in the larger field of intelligence that guides true transformation.

To relinquish the hero role is not to diminish one's contribution. It is to mature into it. It is to recognise that the healing field is co-created, moment by moment, through presence, humility, and relational depth. This is what clients remember—not the brilliance of our analysis, but the steadiness of our being. They remember how we sat with their shame, how we didn't rush to fix it, how we allowed the dignity of their own unfolding.

The healer is not a hero. The healer is a human. And perhaps that is the most powerful medicine of all.

Belonging as Intervention:

The opposite of trauma is not tranquillity—it is belonging. In a world increasingly attentive to biochemical imbalances, genetic predispositions, and individual psychology, we have underestimated the therapeutic force of *being welcomed without condition.* A growing body of research across disciplines—from psychiatry to anthropology—points toward what many Indigenous cultures and community-based traditions have always known: that healing does not occur in isolation. It happens in the presence of others, through *recognition, affirmation, and inclusion.* Belonging, far from being a sentimental ideal, is emerging as one of the most potent determinants of mental, emotional, and physiological wellbeing.

At the physiological level, the need for belonging is not abstract—it is wired into our neurology. Human nervous systems are designed to seek safety in connection. Stephen Porges' Polyvagal Theory reveals that our vagus nerve, which governs the regulation of stress, is attuned to cues of social safety: eye contact, vocal tone, facial expression, presence. When we feel excluded—whether overtly through discrimination or subtly through cultural dissonance—our nervous systems interpret this as danger. The body does not distinguish between the rejection of a tribe and the threat of a predator. *Alienation activates survival responses.* Chronic stress, inflammation, hypervigilance, and even autoimmune conditions often arise not solely from internal pathology but from persistent experiences of not being safe to be oneself.

This is especially relevant when working with individuals whose identities have been marginalised by dominant systems—whether through race, gender, sexuality, neurodivergence, class, or cultural background. Too often, therapeutic models assume a neutral, universal subject. Yet the absence of cultural attunement is not neutrality—it is erasure. When a practitioner fails to acknowledge the lived experience of, say, a queer migrant of colour navigating intergenerational trauma and systemic exclusion, they inadvertently reinforce the very stressors they seek to treat. The therapeutic space becomes yet another site of surveillance and misrecognition, rather than a sanctuary.

Belonging must therefore be understood not as an emotional state alone, but as an *intervention.* It is not an accessory to therapy; it is therapy. Inclusion—when deeply practised—has the power to reorganise a person's relationship to themselves and the world. When someone feels genuinely seen in their specificity, their story begins to reorganise. Shame dissolves. Defensive adaptations soften. The need for hypervigilant self-monitoring decreases. In its place, an internal posture of safety can emerge—not because the person has learned to regulate in isolation, but because their body no longer expects threat in every room they enter.

This is not a theoretical proposition. It is measurable. Studies on the health impacts of discrimination show clear correlations between perceived social exclusion and elevated cortisol, increased risk of cardiovascular disease, and accelerated cellular ageing. Conversely, research into protective factors for mental health repeatedly identifies *community, identity affirmation, and cultural safety* as foundational. For instance, youth who identify as LGBTQ+ but have access to affirming environments—such as schools that respect their pronouns or families that validate their orientation—report significantly lower rates of depression, suicidality, and substance misuse. The protective factor is not internal resilience alone. It is *relational coherence*—the feeling of being mirrored accurately and lovingly in the eyes of others.

This insight invites a reframing of what we consider healing work. It is not enough to provide good technique or evidence-based interventions if the relational field is implicitly invalidating. Cultural safety, a concept developed in New Zealand within Māori healthcare settings, offers a more expansive standard than cultural competence. It demands that practitioners not only understand difference, but actively dismantle power imbalances and reorient practice toward equity. It is not about knowing everything—it is about being willing to ask, to listen, to centre the client's reality as primary. *Power is not neutral in the healing process—it must be negotiated with humility.*

To understand belonging as medicine is also to recognise how its absence—structural and symbolic—creates illness. Poverty is not only material deprivation; it is social exclusion. Racism is not only a psychological wound; it is a chronic stressor that shortens life expectancy. Ableism, when internalised, leads to self-erasure. In each of these, the fundamental injury is not that the person is different, but that their difference is treated as defect. It is the erosion of place. Healing, then, is not the erasure of that difference but the *restoration of rightful place.* The work is not to make someone fit—but to make space sacred enough to hold all that they are.

Modern clinical settings are only beginning to account for this. Group therapy, peer support networks, and community-based healing initiatives—especially those led by people from within the community—are essential counterbalances to individualised care models. But the danger remains that such practices become tokenised, adjuncts to a biomedical model that still privileges white, Western norms. If we are to take belonging seriously, it must be embedded at every level of care—from intake forms to diagnostic criteria, from practitioner training to institutional policy.

The implications extend beyond therapy. Workplaces, schools, spiritual communities, and public institutions all have the potential to either buffer or intensify stress through the degree of safety they afford. Belonging, unlike happiness or relaxation, is not a private feeling. It is a shared space. The health of a person cannot be separated from the health of the environments in which they live. This is why a supplement will not undo the effects of racist policing. Why mindfulness cannot compensate for exclusionary education. Why a probiotic cannot repair the stress of being misgendered at work. These interventions may help—but only if embedded in a field of relational justice.

This also challenges the idea that identity politics is somehow peripheral to health. On the contrary, identity affirmation is a form of care. When a Black client sees a Black therapist, or a neurodivergent child is taught by someone who shares their sensory reality, or a trans person is able to access healthcare without having to explain or justify their existence, the healing effect is not symbolic. It is somatic. The nervous system recognises: *I belong here.* I am not a problem to be solved. I am someone whose life matters.

It is tempting, especially in an individualistic society, to seek solutions that are scalable, private, and commodifiable. Supplements, apps, self-help routines—these are seductive because they do not require structural change. But as long as our interventions remain skin-deep, the root of the wound—disconnection, dislocation, dehumanisation—remains untouched. Belonging is slower. It demands relationship, repair, and reciprocity. But it is precisely this slowness, this depth, that makes it potent. *What is broken in relationship can only be healed in relationship.*

There is a growing movement within integrative medicine and trauma-informed care to honour this truth. Models such as community acupuncture, peer-led support circles, decolonised wellness, and ancestral healing practices are not merely "alternatives"—they are returns. They reassert the ancient truth that *we do not heal alone.* The body knows this. The heart knows this. And the science is catching up.

Belonging is not a luxury. It is the substrate of healing. A nervous system can be regulated, a diet optimised, a mind trained—but without a felt sense of place, safety, and affirmation, the foundation remains unstable. To create cultures of healing, we must move beyond the question of what works, and ask instead: *for whom?* In what context? At what cost? And are we willing to make room—not only for the wounded, but for the whole of who they are?

Until we do, no intervention—however advanced—will be enough. But when we do, when we anchor our healing practices in *belonging as intervention*, we create not just better outcomes, but *better worlds.*

Chapter 10
Becoming the Medicine

In a world enthralled by speed, saturated with distractions, and driven by endless consumption, the most defiant act is not simply knowing better—it is living otherwise. Integration is the discipline of embodying what we already understand. It is the line that divides the overfilled mind from the liberated body, the well-informed from the genuinely well. Here, we begin at what might seem like the end—where insight alone loses its sufficiency, and the journey demands something else: repetition, rhythm, and return. Knowledge, in itself, is not the prize. Embodiment is.

We are steeped in a culture hooked on insight. From podcasts and bestselling self-help to sleek infographics and pop-psychology seminars, the modern seeker can access more mental health vocabulary than most therapists could have dreamt of fifty years ago. Trauma, regulation, mindfulness, attachment—these are no longer niche terms. Yet fluency is not the same as integration. To speak of "boundaries" does not mean one can hold them. To memorise the polyvagal ladder is not to climb it when under duress. Over-intellectualised healing carries a quiet arrogance: mistaking clarity of thought for change at the cellular level. The body is unmoved by theory; it learns only through what is practised—again and again, especially when stress presses in.

Integration is no abstract idea—it is a choreography. The nervous system recalibrates not through singular flashes of realisation, but through repeated contact with safety, slowness, and coherence. Healing must be rehearsed until it becomes second nature. This is why rituals, somatic exercises, rest disciplines, and micro-boundaries outweigh any standalone insight. True transformation seldom strikes like lightning. More often, it is a subtle re-patterning—a quiet tuning of our inner rhythms until life begins to hum with a wiser undertone. To "become the medicine" is not to have conquered the concepts within these pages, but to let their values live in your breath, your posture, your presence, your choices—especially in unobserved moments.

And yet, integration cannot be standardised. No one-size-fits-all protocol exists for healing. The medicine your body needs must be pieced together from what resonates with your history, your nervous system, your context. This chapter sketches a framework for your own healing mandala—a map that gathers the threads of your learnings into something you can actually live by. Not a rigid prescription, but a living guide grounded in curiosity and consistency. Ask yourself: What rhythms bring you back to balance? Which rituals keep you anchored? Which thoughts unravel you? What spaces stoke your distress? Which people restore you? Healing begins when these questions no longer float in the abstract, but actively shape the way you move through your days.

This is not a neat conclusion. It is a threshold. The pivot from "What else can I learn?" to "What am I actually living?" For insight to matter, it must find its way into your habits, your relationships, and your physical environments—it must be metabolised. To know the principles but persist in the same dysregulating patterns is not a failure of willpower; it is a failure in the architecture of integration. Real integration works with the truth of the nervous system: change happens slowly, cyclically, sometimes awkwardly. Which is why this chapter offers the spiral path—a healing model that discards straight-line progress in favour of recurrence. In this light, setbacks are not evidence of failure but invitations to return—this time with more softness, better information, deeper humility. We loop not from brokenness, but from the whole-body process of learning.

The fantasy of linear self-improvement is tempting. It flatters the ego, offers a sense of mastery. But genuine healing honours the psyche's seasons. Regressions can be reorganisations in disguise. Pauses can be gestations. A plateau may be the body's way of letting change settle, as silt sinks in still water. Cyclical growth is not a sign of inefficiency—it is fidelity to how nature itself regenerates, as opposed to the extractive tempo of productivity culture.

To live by rhythm instead of rush, to prize process over performance, is an act of quiet defiance. And so this chapter lands here: integration is both personal and political. Every person who chooses self-regulation over self-abandonment, presence over dissociation, coherence over chaos, participates in a subtle revolution. Healing is not a private indulgence—it is a relational offering. What the world needs now is not a proliferation of experts, but an abundance of embodied people—those who move steadily, carry their values in their very bearing, and generate safety simply by being congruent. To become the medicine is to become a presence others feel before they can name it.

This is the revolution that leaves no banners, only atmospheres. It unfolds not in dramatic gestures but in the texture of your mornings, the cadence of your breath, the pause before your reaction, the reverence you give to rest. It is the gentle sabotage of inherited urgency, of over-functioning without feeling, of the comfortable numbness that passes for normal. Perfection is not the requirement; sincerity is. You are not tasked with fixing the world, but with refusing to recreate, within your own body, the very conditions from which the world is trying to recover. Once healing becomes embodied, it stops being content and turns into conduct—and from there, it ripples outward.

This is not closure. It is an opening, now inside you. An invitation to be a pattern-interrupter, a rhythm-restorer, a coherent force in a fragmented culture. The way ahead will not always be obvious, but clarity tends to grow each time you pause, breathe, return to what you know, and put your values into practice. At its core, integration is not the crossing of a finish line—it is the slow building of trust with yourself.

So this is an emergence, not an ending. The crossing from learning into living. From theory into tissue. From ideas into action. The work that follows is rarely glamorous, but it is sacred. May you become the medicine you sought. May your healing stand as a living presence that heals others. And may your integration ripple into the rooms, the relationships, and the systems that have forgotten how to breathe—until, body by body, we remember.

Knowledge is Not the Goal—Embodiment Is:

The modern wellness landscape is saturated with information. Neuroplasticity, vagus nerve toning, trauma-informed care, breathwork protocols—once esoteric, these concepts now populate casual conversations, wellness apps, and corporate workshops. And yet, for all our increasing fluency, rates of burnout, anxiety, and disconnection continue to rise. The problem is not lack of knowledge. The problem is *disembodiment.* We have become collectors of insight and spectators to our own awareness, rather than practitioners of change. What's missing is not understanding, but *integration.* The body doesn't heal because it knows something. It heals because it *practises* something. Again and again. Wisdom, in the context of chronic stress and sustainable healing, is not cognitive—it is rhythmic.

To embody a truth means to have rehearsed it until it becomes instinctual. It means that under duress, your system doesn't reach for the trauma-conditioned reaction, but for the newly patterned one—automatically, not just theoretically. This is what separates a regulated person from a merely informed one. Many people can explain their attachment style, identify the neural correlates of their stress, and name the legacy burdens they inherited from family systems—but freeze when asked to actually set a boundary, say no, pause before reacting, or rest without guilt. That dissonance is not failure. It's simply the gap between insight and embodiment—and it's a gap that cannot be bridged through thinking alone.

The cognitive revolution of the 20th century framed healing as a shift in beliefs, thoughts, and perceptions. And while cognitive reframing has its place, particularly in trauma work, it is insufficient for nervous system repair. You can believe you are safe and still feel terrified. You can tell yourself you're worthy and still flinch at praise. The body has its own memory, and it speaks in sensation, posture, breath, and pacing. To reach it, you must *speak its language*: repetition, rhythm, and return.

Repetition is not redundancy—it is how the nervous system learns. A regulated body does not result from a singular moment of clarity but from consistent micro-decisions repeated until they create new neural pathways. The healing effect of breathwork, for instance, does not lie in a single exhale but in the daily *practice* of slowing the breath—even on days when it feels boring, mechanical, or frustrating. The same goes for meditation, movement, somatic tracking, and rest hygiene. In embodied healing, *boring is sacred.* It signals that you're engaging with nervous system repair on its terms, not on the dopamine-driven terms of novelty.

Rhythm is the architecture of safety. The body finds safety in predictability—not in rigidity, but in reliable cycles. Infants regulate through the rhythm of heartbeat and voice; adults are no different. When we establish predictable, body-based rhythms—morning rituals, sleep cues, mealtime stillness, walking without devices—we offer the nervous system the conditions to downshift from hypervigilance. This is why trauma recovery often begins with rhythm before it moves into meaning. Dr Bruce Perry, among others, has shown how rhythmic interventions—such as drumming, rocking, chanting—can recalibrate dysregulated systems faster than verbal insight. This is not regression; it is evolutionary biology. Rhythm precedes language in development, and it remains the mother tongue of embodied healing.

Return is where healing solidifies. The return is the practice of re-orienting to what you already know, especially when you've forgotten it. It is not a sign of failure to revisit a lesson or re-engage a practice. It is a mark of maturity. Western culture celebrates novelty and mastery; it sneers at return as if it signals backsliding. But the nervous system is not linear. It learns like a spiral—repeating themes at greater depth with each turn. Embodiment respects this spiral. It expects that you will forget, and it gently directs you back. Again and again. This is not inefficiency—it is fidelity to how humans *actually* change.

To operationalise embodiment, we must shift from thinking about healing as a performance to experiencing it as a *rehearsal.* There is no final, flawless state to attain. There is only increasing attunement—practising the breath until it becomes your anchor, rehearsing rest until it no longer registers as laziness, choosing slowness until it feels like alignment rather than avoidance. Healing becomes real not when it is spoken with eloquence but when it is enacted with frequency. A nervous system doesn't need poetry—it needs *practice.*

Consider the example of a client who knows all the right words. She can speak eloquently about internal family systems, name her protector parts, even cite relevant neuroscience. But in the moment she receives an upsetting email, her body floods with cortisol, her breathing contracts, and she unconsciously begins doom-scrolling. Insight has not yet become regulation. With guidance, she learns to *pause*, put one hand on her chest, exhale longer than she inhales, and name aloud: "I'm feeling flooded." That single somatic cue—practised daily until it becomes automatic—starts to shift her baseline. Over time, it re-patterns her stress response. Not through conceptual understanding, but through bodily rehearsal. *That* is embodiment.

There is a quiet arrogance in thinking we can think our way into change. Intellectualism can be a defence against intimacy with our body's truth. It allows us to stay clever and distant rather than vulnerable and present. Embodiment asks more of us. It asks that we show up consistently, imperfectly, and with reverence for the body's pace. It asks that we treat boredom as a sign of depth, not detour. It asks that we honour process over performance. And most radically, it invites us to believe that healing is not a summit we reach, but a rhythm we return to.

It's worth noting the wider cultural context here. Capitalism is deeply invested in the myth of instantaneous transformation. It prefers the six-week course to the six-year practice, the before-and-after photo to the during. But embodiment rejects that aesthetic. It's unsexy. It's process-heavy. It doesn't sell as easily. It asks us to slow down, to feel more, to do less with more depth. And yet, it is *the only path* that produces durable change. Any protocol that bypasses repetition, rhythm, and return is unlikely to result in sustainable nervous system shift.

To embody healing is not to be perfectly regulated. It is to become someone who *recovers more quickly*, who returns to centre more often, who trusts the body's signals and acts accordingly. It is not about always being calm—it is about becoming *congruent.* That congruence—when inner experience and outer behaviour align—is the soil in which safety, creativity, and connection can grow.

As you move forward, consider how your insights can be ritualised. What practices need to be repeated, what rhythms restored, what truths returned to? Where are you still seeking novelty instead of deepening your embodiment? The work ahead is not complicated. It is consistent. And that is what makes it powerful. To live what you know—not just to know it—is the real revolution. Let every breath, pause, stretch, and stillness become an act of integration. Let your body be the place where wisdom lives—not as information, but as *frequency*.

Building a Personal Healing Mandala:

At some point in every healing process, a critical shift must occur: from consuming insights to curating your own path. The modern seeker is often overwhelmed not by scarcity of tools but by their abundance. Breathwork, bodywork, boundaries. Mindfulness, movement, medication. With so many practices competing for attention, many individuals remain trapped in what might be called therapeutic limbo—perpetually learning, rarely embodying. What's needed is not more inputs, but more *integration.* Healing cannot remain an abstract intention or a vague collection of helpful ideas. It must become architecture—designed, structured, and personalised. This is the promise of the personal healing mandala: a visual and conceptual map of what keeps you whole.

The word "mandala" originates from Sanskrit, loosely translating as "circle" or "centre." In spiritual traditions across Asia and beyond, it represents wholeness, interconnection, and the cyclical nature of existence. In the context of healing, it offers a compelling alternative to linear models of progress. Instead of imagining your growth as a straight upward climb or checklist of goals, the mandala invites you to think in terms of relationships—between practices, between parts of yourself, between your inner world and your outer commitments. It encourages integration, not escalation. And crucially, it decentralises the idea that healing lives outside of you. A mandala doesn't prescribe; it reflects. It becomes a mirror of what your nervous system actually needs to feel anchored, replenished, and connected.

To begin crafting a personal healing mandala is to ask a deeper question: *What are the non-negotiable conditions under which I function well—not just mentally, but physiologically, relationally, and spiritually?* This is not a list of trendy biohacks. It is an exploration of resonance—what brings your system into coherence. One person may find that 20 minutes of silent sitting resets their cortisol levels better than any supplement. Another may need movement first: shaking, walking, dancing to metabolise stress before reflection becomes possible. Another may discover that safety only lands in the presence of another regulated person—that co-regulation, not solitude, is their foundation. No generic wellness protocol can account for this nuance. But your mandala can.

To build it, begin by selecting four to six domains that feel central to your healing ecology. These might include *rest*, *movement*, *expression*, *nourishment*, *connection*, *silence*, *play*, or *structure*. Each domain becomes a quadrant or segment of your mandala. From there, name one or two *specific, sustainable* practices you can commit to in each. Not the ideal version—the real version. If "rest" is a domain, and you know you can realistically lie down for 10 minutes after lunch rather than scheduling a 90-minute nap, include that. If "expression" is core, and journaling feels forced but voice notes come naturally, record those. The point is not aesthetic—it is *functional*. Your mandala should be livable, not aspirational.

This approach also invites a crucial mindset shift: healing is not what you do *once* when everything crashes. It is what you do *repeatedly* to prevent the crash. The personal healing mandala serves as a compass when you've lost internal orientation. When symptoms reappear, stress mounts, or relationships fray, you no longer need to wonder where to start. You look to your mandala. What haven't you touched in the last few days? Which practice has fallen away? What rhythm has become irregular? Healing becomes a return, not a reinvention. This is not a productivity hack—it is a path of self-responsibility rooted in compassion.

Real-world examples make this tangible. Consider a trauma-informed therapist who carries the weight of others' pain daily. Her mandala includes daily breathwork (regulation), weekly voice coaching (expression), regular peer supervision (connection), a hard stop at 5pm (structure), and a Saturday forest walk without devices (restoration). This is not an indulgence—it is her *infrastructure*.

Without it, burnout is not a risk; it is a certainty. Her healing mandala is both a preventative medicine and a professional necessity.

Contrast that with an activist who experiences chronic fatigue and inflammation. Her mandala looks different: she includes cold showers (stimulation), political journaling (meaning-making), cooking from ancestral recipes (belonging), and bi-weekly dance nights (joy). Each component addresses a different part of her biology and identity. The mandala helps her remember that healing is not passive. It is a creative act of selection and commitment.

This practice also helps to mitigate the paralysis of perfectionism. Many people abandon healing practices because they "don't do them right" or "miss a day." The mandala dissolves this binary. It does not demand that you be perfect every day. It asks that you *remain in relationship* to your healing ecosystem. Miss your meditation? Maybe you return to walking barefoot on the grass. Skip your journaling? You might sing aloud instead. Your mandala becomes flexible without becoming formless. It replaces rigidity with rhythm.

Philosophically, this model also resists the medicalisation of healing. Instead of seeing yourself as a patient under treatment, the mandala casts you as a designer of your own sanctuary. This is not the same as self-optimisation or rugged individualism. You are not trying to "fix" yourself. You are attuning to the environments and actions that create coherence. The healing mandala places agency where it belongs: not in the hands of an expert, but within the relational intelligence of your own body-mind system.

One of the more radical aspects of the mandala model is that it foregrounds *continuity* over crisis. In Western culture, many people only engage with healing when something breaks—when anxiety peaks, a relationship ends, or the body screams. The mandala trains a different muscle. It builds capacity through consistency. It says: don't wait for pain to prompt care. Make care a default condition. As somatic educator Resmaa Menakem puts it, "healing doesn't happen in urgency; it happens in repetition." The mandala is your rehearsal space.

Critically, your mandala is not static. It is meant to evolve. What once nourished you may no longer serve. A practice that was medicinal in one season may become mechanical in another. This is not failure—it is feedback. You revise the mandala accordingly. You stay in dialogue with your needs. Your map updates as your terrain shifts. The integrity of the mandala is not in its permanence but in its *responsiveness*. It reflects who you are *now*, not who you were when you first created it.

For those working in community or leadership roles, the mandala can be a shared practice. Groups can co-create collective healing mandalas that reflect shared values and commitments. Families can draw theirs together, identifying rituals that bring them into synchrony. Teams in high-stress sectors—healthcare, education, activism—can use them to normalise care as culture, not afterthought. Healing becomes relational, not private.

Ultimately, building a personal healing mandala is not a creative exercise. It is a declaration: *I take my coherence seriously.* It affirms that your wellbeing is not a side project—it is the scaffolding for everything else. And in a culture that celebrates busyness, applauds burnout, and pathologises rest, that affirmation is quietly revolutionary. You are not a machine to be optimised. You are a system to be supported. The mandala is your map—and your permission.

The Spiral Path: Healing Is Not Linear:

Most people don't quit healing because it's too hard. They quit because they think they're doing it wrong. One difficult day, one flare-up of symptoms, one old pattern re-emerging, and the conclusion arises with brutal certainty: *I've failed. I'm back where I started.* This belief—quietly corrosive—derives not from truth but from an inherited model of progress that is deeply flawed: the linear ideal. In Western cultural frameworks shaped by industrialism and achievement metrics, growth is expected to be forward-moving, stepwise, and ever-ascending. But healing—true, embodied healing—rarely obeys such rules. It does not unfold like a staircase. It spirals.

The spiral path, as a metaphor for personal transformation, is ancient. Indigenous cosmologies, mystical traditions, and nature-based philosophies have long recognised that life moves in cycles: death and rebirth, waxing and waning, expansion and contraction. These systems understand that development is not a matter of leaving the past behind, but revisiting it from new vantage points. What appears to be repetition is often re-entry at a deeper octave. You are not back at square one—you are encountering old terrain with new tools, new awareness, new nervous system capacity. *This is progress*, even if it doesn't look impressive from the outside.

Contemporary neuroscience lends credence to this view. Trauma, stress conditioning, and attachment wounds are stored in subcortical regions of the brain—areas not accessible through intellect alone. Insight doesn't override pattern. You can understand your triggers perfectly and still feel hijacked by them. Why? Because neural pathways, particularly those reinforced by survival, require repetition and safety to rewire. This means you will likely revisit certain lessons multiple times, each time integrating them a little more. This looping isn't regression. It is *refinement.*

Take, for example, someone healing from hyper-independence—a coping pattern rooted in early relational disappointment. Their early healing work might involve recognising the root of their over-functioning and beginning to ask for help. Later, they may find themselves back in that pattern during a crisis. The untrained mind says, "I'm back where I was." But viewed from the spiral model, something new is happening: they notice the pattern faster, they recover more quickly, and they experience less shame. Their body may still default to familiar wiring, but their *relationship to the pattern* has changed. That is growth. That is progress.

The spiral also protects us from the tyranny of perfectionism. Linear models suggest a clear endpoint—healed, complete, optimised. This endpoint fantasy drives many into cycles of overexertion, unrealistic expectations, and eventual collapse. The spiral refuses this finish-line mentality. It reminds us that *healing is not an event to achieve but a rhythm to inhabit.* It is something we return to, recalibrate within, and re-commit to again and again—not because we're failing, but because we're human.

Therapists and clinicians who embrace the spiral framework report greater retention and resilience in their clients. When setbacks are framed not as failures but as expected revisitations, clients exhibit more compassion toward themselves and more perseverance in their work. This is particularly crucial in somatic and trauma-informed settings, where premature reactivity to "relapse" can derail months of careful nervous system work. Teaching clients to *expect the spiral* changes how they metabolise difficulty. Instead of panicking when grief returns or dissociation reappears, they learn to ask, "What is this here to show me this time?" That inquiry transforms resistance into receptivity.

From a systems perspective, linearity is a symptom of industrial logic. The conveyor belt, the academic ladder, the career path—all are structured around fixed stages and clearly demarcated metrics. But humans, like ecosystems, are complex, dynamic, and recursive. Our inner life is more akin to weather than machinery. It includes seasons. There are winters of contraction, springs of emergence, summers of abundance, and autumns of letting go. No season is more "advanced" than the other. Each is essential. The spiral honours this seasonality. It affirms that sometimes, stillness is growth. Sometimes, staying present with what hurts is more courageous than pushing forward.

There is also an ancestral dimension to the spiral. Many people who undertake deep healing work are not only contending with their personal traumas but also inherited imprints—what epigeneticists call *intergenerational transmission*. Patterns of fear, vigilance, silence, or self-abandonment often originate several generations back. When these patterns re-surface in our lives, we're not merely re-experiencing our own pain—we are processing the residue of familial survival strategies. Healing these layers often means returning to similar emotional ground, each time unravelling a bit more of what was never ours to carry. The spiral thus becomes a way of liberating lineage, not just self.

Importantly, the spiral model does not negate structure or accountability. It does not romanticise being stuck or advocate passive endurance. What it offers is *context*. It helps you track your movement in broader arcs, so you don't mistake a dip for disaster. It invites you to notice patterns, not punish them. If you find yourself revisiting anxiety, you ask: Is this a familiar stressor? Am I more aware of it now? What's different in how I'm responding? These questions shift you from collapse into curiosity, and from shame into skillfulness.

Modern coaching and self-help cultures often weaponise the language of progress. "Level up," "upgrade," "manifest"—all imply a one-way ascent. But genuine healing is not glamorous. It is circular, often messy, and deeply humbling. The spiral reminds us that revisiting grief, confronting fear, or needing support again does not negate how far we've come. If anything, it affirms our willingness to stay engaged with life at depth. Returning is not failure. It is fidelity to the work.

The spiral also aligns with many indigenous and pre-modern timekeeping systems. Unlike the Gregorian calendar, which flattens time into a linear march, cultures such as the Mayan, Vedic, and Dagara conceive of time as cyclical—comprised of repeating phases, energetic tides, and ritual recurrence. In these systems, healing is embedded in the *rhythmic re-encounter* with certain stories, ceremonies, and initiations. You don't graduate from them. You rotate through them, deepening your participation. Repetition is not a flaw in the system—it is how wisdom is transferred across generations.

One practical implication of the spiral model is the value of tracking. Journals, somatic logs, reflective practices—they all help us witness how far we've come when our emotional weather clouds our perspective. By revisiting old entries, we can often see what our nervous systems cannot: we are no longer stuck in the same place. We are circling back, but with more presence, more tools, and more compassion. What looks like stalling is often subtle integration at work.

To teach the spiral model is to offer people permission: to falter, to return, to take rest, to change their mind, to lose and regain faith. It is an invitation to hold their humanity with more tenderness. In a culture obsessed with results, that permission is revolutionary. It allows healing to become what it always wanted to be: not an improvement project, but a practice of remembering what was never broken.

Ultimately, the spiral path challenges not just how we think about healing, but how we think about time, value, and the self. It reframes growth not as a straight road but as a sacred rhythm—one that moves through grief, grace, and grounding again and again. There is no final destination, no trophy for emotional perfection. There is only the deepening—a softening spiral that returns us to ourselves, each time with a little more trust.

Becoming a Quiet Revolution:

Revolutions don't always come with banners, chants, or political slogans. Some arrive quietly—in how we breathe, how we touch, how we listen without needing to fix. In a world programmed for velocity, optimisation, and hyper-individualism, *to slow down, to stay present, to live with intention* is a deeply subversive act. Healing, when practiced not only for personal repair but as a way of inhabiting the world differently, becomes political. Not in the partisan sense, but in the existential sense: a reclamation of how power, attention, and care are distributed. To become the medicine is to stop waiting for a better system and *start embodying the values we wish it would hold.* This is the quiet revolution—one that does not shout but transforms.

Modern culture teaches us to locate healing as a backstage activity—private, personal, and preferably invisible. You go off and "fix yourself" before returning to the stage of life, polished and performing. But genuine healing doesn't tuck itself neatly into margins. It changes how you work, parent, shop, walk, disagree, and relate. It leaks into your language. It tempers your urgency. It makes you question what is truly necessary. And in doing so, it subtly destabilises the assumptions of a culture that equates speed with value and productivity with virtue. *This is not softness. It is structural resistance.*

Consider how slowness functions as a form of disruption. In an economy that profits from your constant engagement, slowing down your consumption—of information, goods, stimulation—is not just a wellness strategy, it's a refusal. It interrupts systems of extraction. It creates friction in a culture that depends on your seamless participation. A person who pauses before reacting, who digests before responding, who sits with discomfort instead of escaping it, is not passive. They are choosing not to feed the momentum of dysfunction. They are reclaiming *agency at the level of nervous system.* Slowness, in this context, is not lethargy—it's *precision.*

Presence, too, is radical. In communities fragmented by overstimulation and digital disembodiment, full attention has become a rare commodity. To give it generously—to your child, your partner, your patient, your colleague—is to offer a kind of holding that cannot be bought or hacked. Presence communicates: *You matter. I am with you. I am not elsewhere in my mind while sitting beside you in body.* This quality of attention is more than psychological—it's physiological. It regulates. It coalesces safety. It allows other people to come into coherence simply by being in your field. In this way, healing is no longer confined to therapeutic rooms. It moves through you, to others, *without even trying.*

This is not abstract. We see it in how a teacher who models calm diffuses classroom chaos more effectively than one who relies on authoritarian control. We see it in healthcare workers who touch with reverence and are remembered years after a procedure not for their technical skill, but for their humanity. We see it in community leaders who hold space for grief instead of rushing to resolution. These are not grand acts. They are deliberate micro-presences that *undo violence at the nervous system level.* In a culture saturated with performance, authenticity is a healing frequency.

To become a quiet revolutionary is not to detach from the world's pain, but to engage it with a different kind of stamina—one rooted in coherence, not adrenaline. It requires us to examine the assumptions we've internalised about urgency, competition, and scarcity. Capitalism's most cunning achievement may be convincing us that if we just try harder, heal faster, or optimise better, we'll finally feel whole. But healing that cooperates with these imperatives only perpetuates the very dis-ease it seeks to resolve. The revolution begins when we stop measuring our progress in metrics inherited from systems that never had our wellness in mind.

Instead, we measure by attunement: Am I responding rather than reacting? Am I treating this moment, this conversation, this body, as worthy of dignity? Am I creating space where others can be more themselves—not less? These are quiet metrics. They don't scale well. They won't earn accolades. But they are how cultures shift—from the inside out.

To embody healing values publicly is also to face resistance. A person who opts out of urgency may be seen as unproductive. A parent who refuses punitive discipline may be accused of being permissive. A practitioner who resists diagnostic labels in favour of contextual narratives may be dismissed as unscientific. These are not trivial tensions. They speak to the cost of alignment. But they also reveal the transformational nature of presence: *it confronts*. It shows up in rooms where dissociation is the norm and says, "We can do this differently." That confrontation is sacred. It makes space for emergence.

Of course, none of this implies perfection. The quiet revolutionary doesn't live in a permanent state of zen. They falter. They snap. They binge the news. They run on autopilot. But their compass is different. When they notice disconnection, they *pause*. When they hurt someone, they *repair*. When they veer into reactivity, they *return*. This return is the revolution: not pretending to be whole, but being committed to returning to wholeness again and again. This rhythm of rupture and repair becomes not just a personal practice, but a communal one.

Healing that ends at the self remains incomplete. The purpose of healing is not self-sufficiency—it is *interconnection*. When your capacity expands, so does your ability to *hold*—emotionally, relationally, and ethically. You become a site of refuge in a world that trains people to brace. This doesn't mean being endlessly available. It means being sovereign enough in your own regulation to support co-regulation without depletion. It means *your presence becomes medicine not because you've mastered anything, but because you are available to life as it is*. That is rare. That is revolutionary.

A quiet revolution also redefines leadership. No longer the charismatic expert or forceful visionary, the healing leader becomes a space-maker. They do not centre themselves. They centre context, culture, and co-creation. They ask questions rather than deliver pronouncements. They protect process over performance. In organisations, they model humane pacing. In families, they model attuned repair. In communities, they model solidarity over saviourism. Their authority comes not from distance or mystique but from *resonance*. We trust them because they are willing to be changed.

This model of leadership is not theoretical. It is emerging across fields—from trauma-informed education to restorative justice circles, from decolonial therapy to embodied activism. These movements are quietly rewriting the operating system of healing. They recognise that transformation is not about extraction or replication. It is about creating cultures of safety, agency, and dignity. And such cultures begin not with policies but with *people who live differently*.

If you have spent time on a personal healing path—unlearning self-abandonment, repairing nervous system ruptures, dismantling inherited beliefs—then you have already been preparing. Not just to feel better, but to *become someone whose way of being challenges the status quo*. That is the arc of integration. Not more techniques, but more *integrity*. Less performance, more presence. Fewer masks, more truth.

The revolution we need now does not march under one banner. It cooks dinner with awareness. It offers eye contact in silence. It pauses when someone is struggling. It slows down the meeting so everyone can catch up. It takes rest without apology. It asks, before acting, "Is this aligned with the world I'm trying to build?" These small acts—repeated, rooted, and relational—are how we rewire the collective.

To become the medicine is not a slogan. It is a lifelong practice of *living in accordance with what you know to be true*. It asks not for performance but participation. It does not demand heroism, only fidelity to a deeper rhythm—one that resists urgency, honours process, and treats everyday life as the soil of transformation. In this way, the personal becomes profoundly political. Not through conquest, but through coherence. Not through noise, but through presence. Not through overthrow, but through return.

And that is what makes it a revolution. Quiet, yes—but nothing short of radical.

Conclusion
The Medicine You've Always Known

Some truths aren't stumbled upon so much as they surface—quietly, insistently—like a familiar scent on the wind after rain, or the slow, tidal pull of breath when the world finally falls silent. Healing belongs to this category. It is not a prize to be claimed, but a homecoming to rhythms that existed long before diagnosis or discourse. To instincts that do not answer to algorithms. To a knowing that never needed certificates. This is not indulgent nostalgia; it is precision. For all our triumphs in medicine, psychology, and systems design, one constant endures: you were born with the capacity to heal.

This chapter does not seek to unveil anything new. It is, instead, a reaffirmation of what has always been present. After chapters thick with frameworks, case studies, and neurobiological rationale, we are not propelled forward so much as brought back—to the realisation that the remedy is not external. It is you. None of the practices offered here were prescriptions in the conventional sense; they were permissions—structured ways of returning to what is instinctive, embodied, profoundly human.

We live in a culture that has taught us to distrust our own inner authority. It has trained us to confuse volume for truth, speed for progress, novelty for wisdom. We have been told we are broken, that repair must be outsourced; that we are deficient and require supplementation; that we are ignorant and must be taught. Too often, these narratives serve the machinery of the system more than the needs of the person. They draw us out of our bodies and into abstractions, out of our communities and into platforms, out of the sacred and into the synthetic. To remember the medicine is to begin reversing this drift.

Information alone is not a cure. Integration is. You could consume an entire library on trauma, somatics, ancestral repair, and stress physiology, yet if your pace remains frantic, your connections hollow, your breath shallow, and your decisions perpetually deferred to external authority—then the healing has not left the page. The body does not transform because the intellect is persuaded. It transforms when safety and coherence are restored—and those grow not from content, but from contact: with oneself, with others, with the living world.

Trusting the body's intelligence is no sentimental gesture. It is a reclamation of fidelity to lived experience. The body has no vocabulary for English, yet it is fluent in rhythm. It signals misalignment long before test results confirm it. It senses grief before words give it shape. It stiffens in the presence of coercion, and loosens in the shelter of attunement. Healing begins when we listen to these signals without smothering them. This kind of listening is not a wellness fad—it is the return of agency.

The same is true in our relationship with the earth. For countless generations, humans co-regulated not only with one another but with the land itself. With the sweep of the seasons. With the sun's slow arc. With cycles of decay and renewal. Healing was never extracted; it was enacted in participation. That ethic has been steadily eroded—not just by the engines of industry, but by the conviction that all solutions must be engineered, that regeneration is something purchased, that ancestral ways are mere relics. Yet the earth requires no invention to be medicinal—it requires reciprocity. And reciprocity is an act of remembering, not of innovation.

Here lies one of healing's enduring paradoxes: it is intensely personal, yet inevitably collective. You cannot truly heal in isolation from the social, political, ecological, and cultural currents that shape you. And yet you cannot afford to wait for those systems to be just before beginning. The integration of what you have read here is not a neat checklist—it is a living, evolving map. One you redraw with every breath taken in awareness, every boundary held, every ritual honoured, every moment you choose not to forsake yourself or others. The map is yours to chart. But the truths beneath it are a common inheritance.

At this point, the question is no longer what more you must learn. It is: What have you always known but been taught to forget? Which practices feel intuitively correct, even without the seal of peer-reviewed approval? Which relationships grant your body that unmistakable sense of home? What ancestral or intuitive knowing have you sidelined in your pursuit of evidence, efficiency, or recognition? This is not a summons to anti-intellectualism—it is a call to root your intellect in a deeper soil of knowing.

The medicine you have always known is not abstract. It is physiological, ecological, relational. It appears in the depth of your exhale. In the patience with which you chew your food. In the steadiness you bring into conflict. In whether your values survive the tyranny of your schedule. These are not incidental details; they are diagnostic. They reveal whether your healing is cosmetic or cellular—whether you are adapting to dysfunction or aligning with your truer coherence.

To live as medicine is not to escape pain, but to hold it with discernment. It is to understand that healing is not a destination, but a continual return. One that life may interrupt but never erase. Every tool in these pages has been offered not as a final answer, but as a compass—and a compass is only useful when it brings you back to your own north.

So here is the invitation, stripped of ornament: cease the endless search, and begin the grounded trust. Not a blind or reckless trust, but one rooted in the body, tempered by discernment. Trust that your body carries wisdom beyond language. Trust that the earth, even wounded, still hums to those who will listen. Trust that the old ways—prayer, rest, touch, ritual, song, story, presence—are not outdated, only obscured. They have not vanished; they are waiting for you to remember.

When you do—when you reclaim them not as relics but as tools—you do more than mend yourself. You step into healing as a way of living. A life that does not require crisis to slow down. A life that allows grief without diagnosis. A life in which strength is redefined—not as the capacity to overpower, but as the clarity to discern. A life that sees personal wellbeing and collective liberation as inseparable.

This chapter does not close the book on the subject. It opens the door to a deeper one—where you are no longer a reader, but a participant. A remembering creature. A custodian of wisdom older than modern medicine, subtler than any algorithm, and more urgent than ever. You are not the patient. You are not the project. You are the medicine. Now—live accordingly.

A lyrical return to the book's opening premise:

The idea that healing lies somewhere outside ourselves—waiting in a pill, a professional, or a perfectly executed protocol—is one of the most tenacious myths of modern life. It's a myth that flatters the machinery of commerce, justifies endless consumption, and keeps individuals chasing, consuming, comparing. But if there is one thing the past century of chronic illness, burnout, and fragmented care has revealed, it is this: *we are not healing because we are not listening.* And what we are failing to hear is not exotic or esoteric. It is ancient, local, and already embedded within us.

This final reflection is not a conclusion, but a turning. A redirection of attention from the external to the internal, from acquisition to attunement. What if the most radical act left is not to seek, but to *remember*? Not to innovate, but to *return*? The premise laid out at the start of this book was deceptively simple: healing has never been external. It does not begin in a protocol or a practitioner's room, but in presence—in the deep biological, cultural, and ecological intelligence that animates the body and binds it to the wider world. That premise now comes full circle, not with answers, but with anchoring.

There is a reason that so many of the world's indigenous and ancestral traditions situate the human being *in relationship* with nature, not above or outside of it. In these cosmologies, healing is not a transaction; it is a *homecoming.* To become well is not to be "fixed" but to *realign*—with the rhythms of the earth, the memory of the ancestors, the wisdom of the body, and the coherence of community. Such traditions do not deny the importance of tools or interventions; they simply refuse to de-centre the most essential truth: that you are not fundamentally broken. You are often *misaligned with what you already know to be true.*

The modern clinical gaze struggles with this. Because what cannot be measured often cannot be trusted. What cannot be patented cannot be marketed. And what is intuitive is too easily dismissed as insufficiently rigorous. But lived experience is a kind of evidence. Not the kind you submit to journals, but the kind that makes you exhale more deeply. Sleep more peacefully. Feel safer in your own skin. The more deeply you inhabit your own body, the less susceptible you become to a culture that profits from your disconnection. *Healing, in this view, is not a service. It is a stance.*

What has been explored in this book—rituals, rest, co-regulation, narrative, belonging, breath, slowness—are not modern inventions. They are, in various forms, part of the human record across time and geography. What makes them radical today is not their novelty, but their refusal to conform to the industrial logic that governs so much of modern life. To take rest seriously in a culture addicted to productivity is an act of resistance. To attune to the needs of the body before checking your phone is a quiet revolution. To prioritise communal safety over individual optimisation is a *return to sanity.*

This does not mean rejecting modern medicine or scientific insight. It means refusing to mistake them for wholeness. It means recognising that the body is not a machine to be tuned, but a *living ecosystem* that must be tended. It means remembering that the mind is not a disembodied command centre, but a participant in a network of emotional, relational, ancestral, and ecological forces. *Healing is what happens when that system re-learns how to listen to itself.*

For those who have spent years accumulating knowledge—books, trainings, certifications, symptom trackers—there comes a point where information no longer heals. Insight without embodiment becomes a kind of paralysis. You can know all the right things and still live in disconnection. You can say all the right words and still feel hollow. What's missing is not more content, but *contact*: with the body, with stillness, with the uncommodified world. This contact is often humble. It does not announce itself. It looks like remembering to eat slowly. To notice the seasons. To speak kindly to yourself not as a self-help strategy, but as a *reverent return to inner relationship.*

Much of what's been marketed as "healing" in recent decades has assumed a posture of lack. That you need something external—more expensive, more advanced, more expert. But what if the medicine you need is not scarce? What if it's *abundant, ancestral, and already in motion within you*? What if your healing has less to do with your next breakthrough and more to do with trusting your quietest knowing?

This orientation is not passive. It requires radical discernment. To trust the body after years of disconnection. To trust nature in the face of synthetic substitutes. To trust relationships that don't optimise your brand but *stabilise your nervous system.* This trust is not naïve; it is hard-won. It is reclaimed, sometimes painfully, through grief and letting go. Through remembering the stories you were told about who you are—and choosing to rewrite them.

The reader who has travelled this far knows: there are no magic solutions here. No five-step fixes. No utopias. What there is instead is the beginning of something more robust: *a practice of remembering that wholeness was never lost—only obscured.* The goal now is not to go back to something simpler, but to go deeper into something *truer.* And that truth often shows up in the quietest places: in the soil, in the breath, in the shared silence between two people who feel safe with each other.

To become well in a culture of disconnection is a profoundly political act—not in the partisan sense, but in the deeper sense of *reclaiming sovereignty over your attention, your rhythms, your choices.* It is to become a site of coherence in a time of fragmentation. Not by broadcasting your healing, but by embodying it—in how you rest, relate, listen, eat, repair, and return. Not by becoming invulnerable, but by *becoming available to what is real.*

So these final words do not instruct you to look further. They ask something much harder: *to trust deeper.* To trust that the signals of the body are not nuisances but messages. That the quiet intelligence of the earth has not disappeared—it has only been drowned out. That ancestral knowledge is not quaint—it is adaptive. That your capacity to live differently was never revoked—it was *merely buried under layers of noise.* This book has been an excavation. What you choose to do with what you uncover is up to you.

And perhaps that is the final medicine: to remember that healing was never about adding more. It was about removing what numbed, distracted, and distorted. *What's left is not emptiness—it is clarity.* And with clarity, the way becomes less about control and more about attunement. You are not separate from the healing you seek. You are not the problem to be solved. You are, and have always been, part of the solution.

Remember that. And begin again.

About the Author

Vivienne Mallory is a holistic medicine scholar and eloquent storyteller with over a decade of apprenticeship in naturopathy, Ayurveda, and Eastern healing traditions. Trained in both clinical naturopathy and subtle-energy therapies, she blends rigorous scientific insight with spiritual eloquence—creating a voice that speaks to both the mind and the soul. She has led healing retreats in the Himalayas and coastal North America, bringing ancient modalities into contemporary contexts. Vivienne's work is informed not only by formal study but by lived experience: she healed herself from burnout and chronic stress through the very methods she now teaches. Healing Beyond Pills is her first full-length book, though her shorter titles—such as "Ritual of Resilience" (forthcoming, Mindful Pages)—have already earned praise for their warmth, clarity, and depth. She lives in Vancouver, BC, and can often be found wandering the forest shoreline, gathering herbs, and mapping the body's hidden languages.

www.ingramcontent.com/pod-product-compliance
Lightning Source LLC
Chambersburg PA
CBHW031345230926
51848CB00002B/386
* 9 7 8 9 3 7 1 7 7 4 3 8 3 *